Mothering *from your* Center

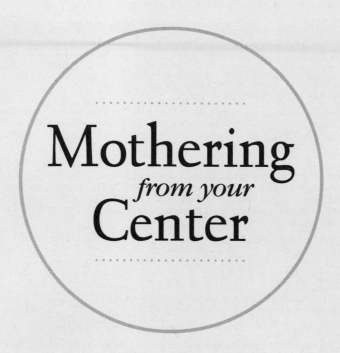

Mothering *from your* Center

Tapping Your Body's Natural Energy for
Pregnancy, Birth, and Parenting

Tami Lynn Kent

ATRIA PAPERBACK
New York London Toronto Sydney New Delhi

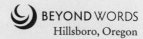 BEYOND WORDS
Hillsboro, Oregon

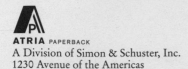
ATRIA PAPERBACK
A Division of Simon & Schuster, Inc.
1230 Avenue of the Americas
New York, NY 10020

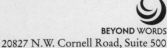
BEYOND WORDS
20827 N.W. Cornell Road, Suite 500
Hillsboro, Oregon 97124-9808
503-531-8700 / 503-531-8773 fax
www.beyondword.com

Managing editor: Lindsay S. Brown
Editor: Jenefer Angell
Copyeditor: Sheila Ashdown
Proofreader: Jade Chan
Design: Devon Smith
Composition: William H. Brunson Typography Services
Author Photo: Shayne Berry, www.shayneberry.com

First Atria Paperback/Beyond Words trade paperback edition February 2013

For more information about special discounts for bulk purchases, please contact Simon & Schuster Special Sales at 1-866-506-1949 or business@simonandschuster.com.

The Simon & Schuster Speakers Bureau can bring authors to your live event. For more information or to book an event, contact the Simon & Schuster Speakers Bureau at 1-866-248-3049 or visit our website at www.simonspeakers.com.

Manufactured in the United States of America

10 9 8 7 6 5 4 3 2 1

Library of Congress Cataloging-in-Publication Data

Kent, Tami Lynn.
    Mothering from your center : tapping your body's natural energy for pregnancy, birth, and parenting / Tami Lynn Kent. — First Atria Paperback/Beyond Words trade paperback edition.
        p.   cm.
    1. Pregnancy—Popular works.   2. Childbirth—Popular works.   3. Motherhood—Popular works.   4. Mind and body—Popular works.   I. Title.
RG551.K46   2013
649'.10242—dc23

2012034848

ISBN 978-1-58270-354-1
ISBN 978-1-4516-6853-7 (eBook)

The corporate mission of Beyond Words Publishing, Inc.: *Inspire to Integrity*

To all who mother—
tending the soul of the children and community.
Thank you for your sacred work.
May you know and love your beauty.

Contents

Dear Reader,

I invite you to journey into the creative center of your female body, to the heart of your mothering. Discover how to tap into your body's natural energy for pregnancy, birth, postpartum healing, and parenting. Find the connection between creative energy flow and the core of your body to reclaim your mothering radiance.

I write this book with deep respect for those who mother; I know how much you do each day in your mothering. My intention is to offer you a resource in this book, a guide to more fully access the beauty of your own center and assist your exquisite mothering path. Living with the spontaneity, lack of predictability, and elusive sense of perfection that tending children brings ultimately reveals the power of keeping ones awareness in the center—this moment where spirit and children reside.

Just like the intense opening that happens in birth, there are times in mothering when your capacity will be stretched to its edges. And just like with birth, the energy in your own center can assist this expansion and offer abundant resources for you and your child.

The nature of mothering is that even when you feel like an expert, your child changes and requires a new set of skills. Again, the energy within your own center is perfectly made for each child and each creation you birth. In fact, accessing the energy of your center ensures that for everything you give, there is all that and more for you to receive.

There is medicine here for you. Even if your starting point for mothering is a difficult childhood or a challenging birth event, the energy that flows through your center can heal and bring forward new ways of being.

This book is not meant to take the place of medical advice or your own intuition.

May you know the power, spirit, and joy of mothering from your center.

mother (mu*th*'er) n. that which gives birth to something, is the origin or source of something, or nurtures in the manner of a mother.

Foreword

My daughter Kate and I sat together on a glorious Saturday in June 2012, poring over the manuscript of *Mothering from Your Center* and looking back over our own twenty-nine years as mother and daughter. Though this foreword is written in Kate's voice, it is a true co-creation. I'm sitting right here with her—and with you.

My mother was doing deliveries, cesareans, and hysterectomies while I was in utero. And from her women's medical practice, my mother—a trailblazer—created a completely new language for women's wisdom. It's a language that in the entire field of medicine barely existed at that time, and it was created while I gestated in the field of the most intense energies of the female pelvic bowl.

"Most modern women embody a masculine pattern of *doing* and *driving* that goes counter to the more feminine, internal, and cyclical nature of the womb," Tami writes. My mother was the epitome of this as she birthed her work on the planet. Her generation witnessed mothers who were limited by the societal prix fixe menu: nurse, teacher, secretary, or mother. Choose one—no substitutions, please. As I write, my mother reminds me, "The biggest burdens for a child are the unlived dreams of their mother." And so, her generation went out to express what their mothers couldn't. They became doctors, lawyers, CEOs, heads of state, and leaders of empires. They wore suits and eschewed anything too feminine: "No frills or high heels for me. I'm being a man, thank you very much. I have no need for those things."

It was when she was pregnant with me that she began the journey of breaking through to her writer's voice, which led to *Women's Bodies, Women's Wisdom* and other books. She didn't think that she could write, and took the proprioceptive writing course because there was no language to describe what she was seeing in her practice. The entire time, she was terrified that she wouldn't be able to fully mother and love a second child, given the demands of her work. She would soothe herself with the knowledge that we were old friends and that I wouldn't even have come to her if I hadn't known what I was getting myself into.

When I was two, my mother left her conventional practice to cofound Women to Women in a big old Victorian house where ten children had been raised. My mother remembers saying to herself, "'Where do women feel the most comfortable and safe? At home.' So we made the old bedrooms into exam rooms and we put couches in all the offices. Women would come into this house and sit on the couches, tell their stories, and sob. We created a safe place for women to share what was truly in their hearts and wombs."

Years later, when I had my first pelvic exam at Women to Women, I burst into tears and simply couldn't stop crying. I, too, had become one of the women who felt safe enough in this womb space to be completely free, and to heal as a result.

The importance of home has been a central theme in my relationship with my mother. And for me, the concept of home has often been synonymous with her. I'm one of the lucky ones whose home has always been safe, warm, and inviting, all because of my mother's fierce "mother bear" instincts about what is most important in life. Home has been a place to seek solace, to be unconditionally loved, and to bring friends who will be embraced with the same open arms in which I'm wrapped when I step through the front door.

My mother still lives in the house in which I grew up. We sit writing this together, in the office where I would often come and lie around after school as a teenager, watching her type away on her computer and research her next book. I have just moved back to Maine and have only recently allowed myself to admit that a significant reason for my coming home is to live near my mom again. (Though she assures me that I hadn't been fooling anyone.)

Tami's *Mothering from Your Center* reminds us of our sacred feminine center, from which all life springs and from which all our creativity radiates. Tami speaks of "wild mothering" as a flow of creative energy that extends mothering "beyond basic caregiving into the making of a soul-filled life." She reminds us that mothering is the most important job in the world. But unlike many of our mothers' generation, she also knows the importance of taking care of ourselves and the importance of helping our children negotiate loss, change, and anger.

As women, we are called to serve our husbands, our partners, our homes, our communities, our careers, our mothers, our friends, and, most of all, our children. Tami's wise writing and my experience of having been raised by a woman who understands this, too, tells us that the best way to serve is to tap into our own deep, wise, wild feminine center. We can access and give expression to the fullness of our dreams as women and mothers. We can model and give permission for our loved ones to tap into their own centers and, eventually, source their lives from their own well of creativity. When we are given permission to live our own truth through our bodies, like I was as a child, we will never go a day without access to the Divine Mother within.

The women (and men) of my generation are able to come home because the women in my mother's generation left home. My mother and her contemporaries swung the pendulum way past where it had been in order to break new ground for women. And they did a damn good job, in my opinion.

What's so beautiful is that now, at the age of twenty-nine, probably a few years out from becoming a mother myself, I have the profound honor of witnessing my mother come home to herself. She's more beautiful, feminine, and receptive than I've ever seen her in my life. The birthing process, it turns out, is ongoing and self-renewing.

My mother told me that we pick our parents. Growing up, when my sister and I would get upset with her, she would tell us that we were more than welcome to go out and pick a different mother. And inevitably we would look around at the other options out there—other women we saw at the grocery store, our friends' mothers, and so on—and we would reluctantly agree that she had been a pretty good choice. The biggest gift you can give a child is your full embodiment of who you truly are. When a mother lives full out from her center—the way I see my mother living these days—it swings the door wide open for her children to do the same—and even more.

I'm deeply grateful to have the wild mother I chose. And when you read and absorb the wisdom in this profoundly touching and helpful book, chances are really good that your child will feel the same way, too!

—Christiane Northrup, MD,
and Kate Northrup

Christiane Northrup, MD, is an ob/gyn physician and author of the *New York Times* bestsellers *Women's Bodies, Women's Wisdom* and *The Wisdom of Menopause.*

Kate Northrup is the author of *Money: A Love Story.*

The Great Mother

One of my boys holds my right arm and has curled it around his body so that this part of me is more his than mine. The baby is on the other side, alternately murmuring to my hand and then turning to nurse at my breast. Back and forth, with eyes closed, he seems to be saying a baby prayer.

I am lying in the family bed, trying to be still so my restless sons will find sleep. Mothering contains countless moments where I am at the mercy of a rhythm other than my own. I feel the restlessness of my own cells rise to the surface, and I resist the urge to get up and disrupt their journey to near-sleep. Instead I focus on the hot evening air and the hot breath of each boy beside me. The resistance in my body releases as I drop my awareness into the beauty of this moment.

Indeed, my left hand feels blessed by this soft baby breath. His murmurs fill my palm like a chant. I wonder if he knows that these hands are my life. I write, mother, and heal with my hands. Thinking back to how it was with him in the belly and to what I see now each time I look into his eyes, I am certain that his addressing of this hand is intentional.

I ponder the essence of the Great Mother and the mothering tasks that fill my days now. The Great Mother is not an example of perfection to measure ourselves against, but rather our collective capacity to exist in the moment, relishing that which sustains us. It is an ability to sit in the fire of our making long enough to see what we have created. We return to our womb, the source of our creative inspiration, so that we may know our mothering gifts. We reclaim the wild part of ourselves and mother from this spontaneous and untamed place. Realigning with the Great Mother means calling spirit down through our mothering.

One does not have to be a mother to access this essence. Every woman who returns to the center of her being to mother her heart-felt creations can call forth the creative essence that is her birthright. By paying attention to the rhythmical cycles of her womb, a woman encounters the Great Mother, the presence of the sacred feminine that infuses all of life. Whether a person is giving birth or living with a sense of expansion that often accompanies the creative process, the Great Mother teaches her how to be with spirit.

I sense, as I always do, the instant my children fall asleep. There is a sudden softening as their breathing deepens. I become giddy, having bridged the place between struggle and breath. No part of me can rest until they do, and I ache with my own wants that resurface as the night settles in. I trace each son's soft skin, smooth as butter.

My heart is torn by two wants. I want to go and walk about the quiet of the house by myself as a woman. I want to stay and linger in the boyish scent of these sleeping children. I am Mama. I am me. I see the boys' small wrists, their small arms. Their throats are open and perfectly smooth. They have small mouths and small bodies. Everything about them seems small when they are sleeping. My baby's mouth will search for a nipple in his sleep. My son will reach until he finds skin. I am their source, and they touch me to find themselves. The sky goes from pink to blue to black. I lie, arms anchored by two sleeping angels, and contemplate the word *surrender*.

Surrender and spirit are words whose meanings are intimately connected. To know this is to know the heart of wild mothering.

Journey into Mothering

Imagine an alchemic fusion that ignites in your center and illuminates your life. This is the mystical pathway of all creation, universally passing through conception, pregnancy, birth, and the many seasons of mothering that make up a lineage of motherhood. Like all epic journeys, it requires a passage into the unknown. We open to this miracle of life, but the timing of conception or birth remains a mystery. With a baby in the womb, we can know his or her gender, but their unique presence will only be discovered day by day in the experiences woven together through time. Even the energy movement that accompanies each soul into life is largely beyond our comprehension. In becoming a mother, we step into the line of mothers that extends through the generations behind us. Through this touch from spirit in the center of ourselves, we begin a process of transformation that reveals who we are and who we will become.

As a women's health physical therapist and energy reader, I have worked with thousands of women to understand the creative potential we carry in our bodies. From this collective wisdom, I made an energetic map of the pelvic bowl—as both a physical structure and profoundly creative space in the female body, the feminine landscape where we gestate and birth our creations. I explored new ways of intentionally engaging this place where spirit meets body in my first book, *Wild Feminine*. Now in this book I apply this knowledge specifically to pregnancy, birth, and mothering.

Though pregnancy and birth bring us back to the center of our bodies, the children we mother continue to call us back to the center of our lives. If we heed this call, back to the center, we not only have more energy upon which to make our mothering but we also contact this beautiful and wild part of our feminine nature. Returning to the center and living from here is what I refer to as "wild mothering" or extending the flow of your creative energy beyond basic caregiving into the making of a soul-filled life.

Within these pages, I have included the essential tools to restore your center and mother from this place. There are resources to holistically heal your body after birthing, both for the initial post-partum phase and the long-term postpartum effects. Based on my background in physical medicine and the practice of Holistic Pelvic Care™ I have developed, I share the information that is vital to caring for your pelvic bowl and restoring your radiant form. I also include groundbreaking energy medicine that I have created for accessing the healing potential of birth, even long after a child is born, and to use this potent creative energy for life. Keep in mind that many of the lessons learned from the physical aspects of pregnancy and birth can be applied to any number of forms of creative completion and evolution, all of which draw upon the energies in a woman's body.

My practice as a healer has taught me that a woman's creative essence provides her with infinite resources. The energy in the creative center can assist the forging of new patterns for mothering as well as new ways of engaging the creative flow. Working in sync with the creative currents that move through the body, mothering and creativity complement one another, energizing rather than depleting as a way of "mothering from the center."

This book is not a call to do more; it is a guide for accessing the potential you already contain. In my practice, I teach women to use energy-sensing tools and centering meditations that I use in my own home to align the energy field for my family. These practices address the real stresses of mothering and transform the experience into a creative practice for cultivating power, spirit, and joy.

By learning to sense the deeper layers of spirit that awaken within your core when you bring a soul into being, you can meet directly with this mystery. Working with your child's birth energy and its connection to your own body will not only assist the birth process but add potency to your mothering. If you have a miscarriage or birth loss, connecting with the spirit of your child will unfold the blessings from this touch to your womb.

And whether or not you have had a child, whether you tend a hearth for yourself or a family, this book will reveal the miracle of your own birth and beginning as well as how to engage your own creative essence. If you have not experienced pregnancy or birth, I invite you to intentionally reclaim your mothering essence. Every woman who returns to the energy potential of her center will find an ancient rhythm for giving life to her dreams.

I have savored this mothering journey myself, giving birth to three sons and one spirit daughter. With these tools to activate my core creativity, I live the experience of a wild motherhood that is attuned to the rhythms within each day and aligned with an inherent flow. This flow brings an intuitive responsiveness that serves me as a creative being as well as the deeper needs of my children. In exploring my capacity for wild mothering, I have never felt more alive, radiant, and connected to the pulse of life.

Though it was through my work and more than a decade of mothering that I learned how to apply this creative essence to living, this book contains all the information I wish I had been given from the moment I said yes to becoming a mother. It is told in my voice, yet the knowledge shared represents the collective voices of the many women whose bodies and energies have graced my women's health practice. Together we learned about the power of the creative current in the female body as a vital resource. I give this to you now, wherever you are in your mothering journey, and invite you to discover the beauty and passion of mothering from your own center.

A Return to the Center

I began my work attending to the physical realm of the female body. However, as a holistic women's health physical therapist, I was most struck by the power of aligning creative energy from the center and witnessing the radiating effects throughout a woman's life. This energy in our centers is related to everything—all that we will make in our lives and all that our soul desires.

All holistic medicine practices have an understanding of energy as chi, the elemental force or spirit that circulates through the body and infuses the cells. Cultivating this essential force that flows in the pelvic bowl is all the more powerful because it is the place where we come into being; it is the spirit door.

It took me a decade of studying the female pelvis to create a framework for comprehending this mystery, but my own intimate knowledge regarding the connection between spirit and form in my body came with a mystical experience of miscarriage.

Prior to my mystical miscarriage, I was still in the process of rebuilding a connection to my own body. This process began with the birth of my first son. But in the days and weeks after he was born, I recognized that everything I had done in preparing for my professional life had taken me outside of my body. I had honed my mental skills in college, graduate school, and my profession as a physical therapist. In my career, I had completed a detailed study of the body and even the pelvic bowl but had not really inhabited this place myself.

Only in my son's birth and the first months of mothering him did I hear the call back to my own center and realize I had been living so long outside this place. Birth required that I come into my center, but then being in the home with my newborn called my attention to the center as well. Returning to this lonely ground, I began to tend it while also tending my young son. It was slow going. It took years of caring for my center and sorting through the accumulation of unmet needs to have enough ground cleared and recovered that I could be sustained by the fertility of my being.

When my first son was two, I had the beginnings of a more organic rhythm for us. With a child in my midst, I no longer had the space to accomplish long lists of objectives each day, and I learned to follow a deeper flow that arises while tending the home fire. I share the story of my physical miscarriage, which occurred in the quiet of our home, in *Wild Feminine*. But I now want to tell the story of the energetic process of my miscarriage, which gave me an intimate understanding of the spirit door and its relationship to the creative center.

The Spirit Door in My Body

It was early summer, and I was still nursing my son. My menstrual period had not yet returned. Though my husband and I were not trying to conceive, and in fact were not sure about having more than one child at this point, I kept feeling as if I were pregnant. One day midsummer, I was taking a shower. My son walked by and said, "Mama, there's a baby in your belly." He was intuiting exactly what I was sensing. I took a pregnancy test: negative.

August came. We went swimming to cool ourselves in the midst of the summer heat. I continued to feel a fullness in my body as if I were pregnant. Then, on a cloudless morning, I awoke with a heavy grief like I had never felt. It was a profound sense of loss that seemingly came out of nowhere. My husband had a work conference, and I remember moving through the day with my son in a surreal way, as if in a dream.

As the day unfolded, I felt compelled to go to Breitenbush, a spiritual retreat center nestled among wilderness hot springs on the edge of the Cascade mountain range a few hours southeast of my home. I called to make a day reservation for us. No luck. Breitenbush was full. I put my son in the car anyway and began to drive, propelled by an invisible force. I prayed, *Please let a space open for us*. I figured I would beg if I had to. It did not feel like there was an option.

I drove in a dreamlike state for about an hour and then called Breitenbush again. They had received a cancellation and had a space available for two. The thought that I would not have to plead to be allowed in while feeling so vulnerable was a relief. I began to cry; I did not know why I was crying other than I felt as if I were being held while experiencing the deepest grief of my life.

When we arrived, we parked on a gravel road beneath towering firs and made our way to the check-in and then to a set of pools surrounded by soft ferns and ancient stones. Entering the warm water with my son, I immediately felt a sharp ache on my right side. I had been working with energy medicine for a few years by this point, and so I began to work with the energy of my body. I realized that the level of intensity I was feeling would require assistance. In an unusual surrender of my high-achieving

"I can do it myself" persona, I cried out to spirit, *I'm going to need help with this.*

Just then, three women came through the trees on the path above the pool. "Are any of you healers?" I called to them.

One of them answered, "We all are."

Well, of course; this was Breitenbush, after all. But I have thought of them since as three goddesses. One entered the water and sat near my head with her large pendulous breasts. Having not been breastfed myself, there was comfort in laying my head against her bare chest.

The second goddess held the center of my body and pelvis as I lay back on the water, and the third one sat with my son. I marvel now at the trust I placed in these women, whom I had never met before. My nature was fiercely independent; I had learned to do things for myself rather than trust others. In this moment, I opened myself completely, held by the same loving presence that had guided me here.

The pain in my side became stronger, and I began to breathe heavily. Having been through one birth experience already, I was prepared to meet what was coming. I realized I was traveling to the spirit door to birth something. Though my logical mind could not comprehend or contain what was happening, my body knew what to do. Now that I was held by the three goddesses, I focused on the ripples coming through my body.

With birth, a physical and an energetic door opens. We talk about the physical opening and the dilation of the womb, but our lack of energy understanding has numbed our ability to sense the energetic opening that occurs. I lay upon the water, the women holding me, and felt the physical contractions and the speed of my breath slowly opening the energy field of the spirit door.

At the point of full surrender and expansion, I saw, with my inner vision, something rise from my body. To my mind's eye, it looked like a goddess I had seen in drawings from India. She was covered in silks and jewels, a radiant vision bathed in red. I watched her lift toward the sky. As she rose, I heard, *The feminine can never be destroyed.* It took me many more years of traveling this life to understand that those intense words contained a profound message of hope: no matter what we might see or feel or experience, the beauty, comfort, and salve of the feminine is there for us always—if we remember our feminine way.

The sacred image lifted and dispersed into the air. My breathing became softer, and I remembered where I was. My body no longer shuddered with contractions, and I began to move with intention. I turned my head to find my son, who was playing contentedly at the side of the pool with one of the goddesses. The other two women continued to anchor me as I came back to myself.

A Message from Spirit to Body

When the experience settled, we began to talk. The woman who sat with my son shared that her twenty-year-old son had died in a tragic car accident the week before. Tears filled her eyes; sitting with my son and witnessing this event had been medicine for her.

It was a profound healing for me as well, but to be honest, I was not sure what had happened or why. I still ponder its mystery. I do know that about five days later I still felt pregnant. I took a pregnancy test, and this time the test was positive. Then my son walked by the shower again and said, "Mama, there's no baby in your belly."

I answered, "Yes, there is, honey. Remember before when you said there was a baby? Well, now it seems there is."

Speaking logically is at odds with the mystery children live in. He simply answered, "No, Mama, there's no baby."

The next morning, I awoke bleeding and would later miscarry a tiny placenta and hint of a being in our home.

Perhaps the positive pregnancy test was a signal to help me understand that I had truly birthed—that my womb was involved in connecting with this tremendous experience. It was the first time I had come into conscious contact with this spirit door in my body or comprehended the depth of its capacity. Though I had birthed before, I did not yet have the ability to sense energy enough to know what was happening in my own center. And the burden of my bodily grief, previously stored but inaccessible, was lifted by this visitation from spirit. My creative field—my wild feminine landscape—felt lighter and more alive than ever before. The August light shimmered. I could see and sense more of the energy potential that was always there, the energy of everything.

I asked my spirit daughter how I might honor her. In response, I saw her sitting with thousands of souls spread out as far as I could see. *Teach women to know the beauty of their bodies and to celebrate the feminine within themselves.* In that moment, I understood a profound truth. If the mothers knew their own bodies as sacred, then the children—and each one of us—could come into the womb as a sacred space. In this way, we might remember our sacredness from the very beginning and bring this potential to the center of our lives.

ONE

Becoming a Mother

Mothering is a hands-on creative process that can be tended and shaped like any creation. Spirit is calling you to mother something born of your own essence and experience. This master-work of your mothering, your *motherpiece*, is essential. As you grow into your motherhood, your way of being will change. These evolutions inspire the palate for creations and additions to your motherpiece. Mothering becomes an inspired process for giving expression to your creative essence.

In my women's health practice, I have learned to read the energy patterns of the pelvic bowl, including organ energies and energy flow that change with a woman's creative cycle. Pregnancy has a distinct sense of energetic fullness. The energy gathers to sustain a new life. Three times I have felt the fullness of pregnancy energy in the pelvis of women who have come to see me, only to find that they were not yet pregnant. In each case, the woman had a menstrual period and then became pregnant on her next ovulation cycle. Two of the women were actively trying to conceive, and in one case it was a happy surprise.

I am intrigued by this sense of energetic fullness in a woman's pelvis, the way the energy of pregnancy is palpable before an actual pregnancy. A colleague who is an acupuncturist relayed a concept from one of her Oriental medicine teachers: the energy of conception is thought to occur three months prior to a physical conception. For a Western mind, this challenges our understanding of conception as only a physical process. But the more I learn about the relationship between the energy flow and subsequent response in the physical field, the more this idea of conception energy makes sense.

I ponder my personal experience with conception. With each of our sons, there was a conscious yes, a point where my husband and I made a decision or accepted the potential of pregnancy about three months prior to the physical manifestation. But what about accidental pregnancies? Or women who do everything they can to conceive but to no avail? Conception and the embodiment of a new soul is one of life's great mysteries. Energetically, for any creation we make, we hold the essence in the center of our body. When I am writing a book, I feel pregnant with the creative energy that will infuse my creation. Working with the energy in the center, a woman can consciously cultivate what she creates in every aspect of her life.

When, then, does one become a mother? Is it marked by conception, pregnancy, birth, or adopting a child? Rather than a certain beginning point, I think of motherhood as a process of becoming— much like life is made by living. After a decade of mothering, I know significantly more than when I began. I thank my oldest son for being "my first pancake" and coming into a new set of parents. Besides tending a child and working with your creative essence, becoming a mother also requires addressing your mothering lineage.

Most of the women I see in my practice have "mother issues," meaning that they struggle with various aspects of how they were mothered or the relationship with their mother. Though there can be "father issues" for women as well, becoming a mother means stepping into the lineage of motherhood: renegotiating the lines that define it and making your own mothering imprint.

Mothering as a Spiritual Path

Mothering is a true spiritual path in that it will expand your spirit, make painfully visible your personal limitations, and bring some of the greatest heart-opening moments of bliss—sometimes all in one day. When you bring forth something new from the center of your being—giving life to a child or a creative manifestation such as a work of art—there is an intensity in this process, like the heat of a kiln as it fires clay. This creative intensity is generated by the immense task of nurturing a new soul while simultaneously becoming aware of one's inadequacies to do so.

I stepped into motherhood after a full-tilt decade of driving ambition that took me through my professional education and into my career as a physical therapist. This all came to a screeching halt with the infant pace of my first son. Instead of the high velocity I had become accustomed to, each day in the first year of tending my son stretched out in long swaths of time, with little structure and the infinite nonlinear caregiving tasks. Like many mothers who find themselves in this position, I was both amazed by my son's beauty and confounded by my lack of preparation for this shift in how I lived. My body pulsed with the current of the external world and the rapid pace of its culture; yet now my focus was my home and my baby, who began quite literally with tiny movements that barely reached outside his parents' arms or the bed where we lay.

To mother my first son, and eventually three, from a more whole place, I went to the deeper currents of the spirit realm. I learned how to care for my wild feminine energy, to supply the stores needed for bringing my children forth and tending them as well as my women's health practice and writing. My guidance for mothering and creative direction came from being present in my own center. In my work and my life, I have found that if a woman attunes to her center, her body contains vast information for cultivating all she tends. By developing my family life and work practice from the organic flow of spirit energy that moves from within, I hope to teach my children to attune to their own creative centers as well. I want my sons to witness that by opening ourselves to the possibility in each moment, we are most likely to encounter the sacred in the midst of living an awakened life. By meeting spirit in this way, we tend to its presence in our lives naturally, finding a deep satisfaction as we do so.

The Mother Place

The uterus is our direct connection to the Great Mother, drawing in the raw potential to manifest and tend our creations. In *Wild Feminine*, I shared my experiences of working with the pelvic bowl and the surprising realization that women are typically lacking presence in their creative core. Modern women are generally unaware of how to access their own powerful root source of creative and feminine energies, and this contributes to a general ambivalence about mothering. Yet mothering calls us directly back to the home and the center of ourselves. Learning to access these root energies for our mothering enables us to harness this core creative essence for making a soulful life with our children.

The womb is a sacred place, whether we carry children there or cultivate our best creative work. Forming a relationship with the womb and realigning with this place of mothering are essential to activating the creative potential in all that we do. Ponder your own relationship with your womb and mothering essence with the following exercise.

Exercise: Creative Essence Meditation

1. *Imagine your creative essence, your mothering capacity.* What does it look like? How does it feel? Where do you access it within your body?

2. *Reflect upon how you are presently using your female energy to create or sustain something in your daily life.* What inner rhythms or guidance are you following? Are you nourishing yourself as a part of your mothering? Is this how you desire to use your creative essence?

3. *Ponder your creative desires.* What do you love? How does your creative essence seek expression? How can this connect to your mothering?

4. *Imagine a sacred place in the wild, or find a place to sit where you are directly in contact with the earth.* Let your center respond to this vision or earth connection. What makes your creative energy come alive? How does your body feel when you access this potential?

5. *Remind yourself to connect regularly with your own creative wellspring.* Garden, sing, or take an art or movement class. You can even shape your whole day from this inner creative current. Let your mothering come from within and take note of the beauty that arises.

Practicing Presence and Tending to Spirit

Within each day and every creative cycle, there is an energy current we can pay attention to and even synchronize with. In doing so, we discover our ability to tend spirit while also attending to the details of living. Trying to make sense of my days with my children, I reached beyond the idea of a schedule based solely on time. Instead of a rigid structure, our schedule was made from the flow of each day. Any agenda or item on the to-do list could easily shift when a child became tired or ill or required extra comfort. Our rhythm also shifted from season to season or as we had more children and our family needs changed. Together we moved through creative cycles large and small that evolved as they transitioned from babies to toddlers and to increasingly independent—but still profoundly connected—school-age children and beyond.

Practicing presence, by noticing the movement that infuses a moment or a particular aspect of life, we receive a direct connection with the divine. Moving away from outer distractions and instead dropping into pure presence as mothers, we can access the greater energies that are always there to inspire and sustain us. We begin to witness our blessings as part of our daily routine, nourishing the soul just as naturally as we eat or breathe.

What new rhythms have come in the process of mothering?
How has your way of being been reinspired?

Embracing the Shadow

Accepting the path of motherhood will not simply bring you to your place of joy or connection with spirit; rather, it often will reveal where you have blocks. Like all spiritual journeys, the challenges you encounter will show the psychic debris that has accumulated in your energetic field.

With its rigorous and prolonged period of demands, mothering taxes the body, mind, and soul in a manner similar to a grueling meditation regimen. On a spiritual retreat, participants often awaken in the early hours of the morning to meditate, placing the body in a zone of discomfort designed to clarify the spirit. Mothering does the same. The children you tend will assist you in meeting your shadow and finding the obstacles that limit your spiritual growth.

In this process of transformation, the intensity of mothering reveals a woman's roughest edges. I thought of myself as a composed and compassionate person until I became a mother. Then I realized that my thoughtful demeanor actually arose from my ability to control many aspects of my life. Similar to the spiritual seekers who live a comfortable life but then are surprised by the difficult feelings they encounter on a spiritual retreat, I came face to face with my own internal hungers. By entering the often nonlinear path of mothering, where my time was organized by the home-based needs of my infant, I had no choice but to face the stored energies and dormant needs of my spirit, which I had previously managed to ignore.

In mothering from the center, we can also encounter a more authentic self. Living and growing with children, who live entirely in the present moment, fosters authenticity. Tending children, your world slows just enough to invite a return to the core, which allows for more authentic ways of being. Be willing to meet the places where your spirit has gone hungry, and tend yourself as well. Mothering from this central place—from where your children arise—takes you to the heart of what matters and reconnects you with the essence of life.

What mystery does mothering invite you toward?

How are you challenged and blessed by the spiritual journey of mothering?

How can you embrace a particular challenge to receive the blessing?

Traversing the Wild Feminine Landscape

The *wild feminine landscape* is the term I use to refer to the energetic and physical creative range within the female body. In referencing this creative center, I intentionally chose words that evoke the resonance between the female body and the earth as the place where we can cultivate our own creative potential.

I have come to know this place in my work with the female body as a women's health physical therapist. My profession embodies the best preventative medicine for women's health, yet this medicine is hardly known. Women's health physical therapy has some amazing physical medicine tools to address and resolve pelvic problems like pain or prolapse (when the uterus or bladder fall toward the vaginal opening) as well as to augment postpartum healing, but the model for women's healthcare is not yet preventative or holistic in its general approach.

One of the essential women's health physical therapy tools is an internal vaginal massage, which rebalances pelvic muscles and fascia. Fascia is a sheath layer that wraps around the organs and muscles, providing an internal elastic support system. Birthing or even a hard fall to the pelvis can set up tension patterns or adhesions in the fascial layer, disrupting pelvic health. Aligning the fascia through vaginal massage (also termed *internal myofascial release*), restores the full engagement of the pelvic muscles, proper alignment of the pelvic organs, sexual vibrance, and the energy flow of the core.

By enhancing the core flow, vaginal massage brings greater vivacity to the female body and ought to be a basic part of women's healthcare. The health in the pelvic bowl affects many aspects, from how a woman's body supports her to how much pleasure she can access. In fact, while I have used vaginal massage to alleviate a myriad of pelvic symptoms, women have also reported increased vitality, improved libido, and a more dynamic feeling within. This core energy flow also determines a woman's creative capacity.

After working in the pelvic bowl with thousands of women, I see these core physical and energetic patterns as a filter through which we perceive and manifest our creative lives. We inherit many of these patterns from our lineage and life experience, but they can interact with and be shaped by ways that support more creative abundance and flow. By exploring the physical, energetic, and spiritual aspects of our female form, we discover the lines that define our creative range. We also find places to restore or expand this range so that it better serves our creative lives as women and mothers (rather than living with only what we were given).

The physical body, including the pelvic bowl, contains your physical patterns and embodied forms that define your creative capacity and fertility. Around the physical core is the energy of the pelvic organs. In this physical and energetic meeting place, there are creative patterns and ways of using energy that influence all you create as a woman. Physical alignment in the pelvic bowl supports energy flow; energetic alignment enhances physical vitality. The more you understand how to work with this vibrance of your pelvic bowl, the more you gain your full range of creative potential.

Delving into the mystical, we must remember our female bodies as a doorway to the divine, where life enters. In the creation of a child, a spirit enters from the spiritual realm. Energy gathers in the womb, and a physical body is made. Here is where spirit comes into form, where spirit becomes embodied. Alignment in the center, both physical and energetic alignment, means more flow, an expanded creative potential, and access to the greater energy and resources of spirit. Working with

Wild Feminine Landscape

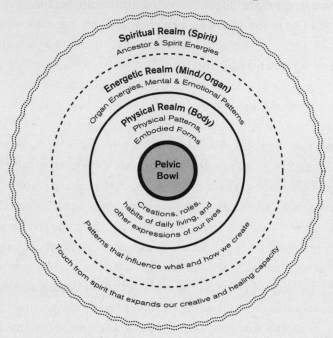

Physical tension and energetic blocks in the pelvic bowl limit core vitality and energy flow. Conversely, physical alignment and balanced energy patterns create robust health and the potential for greater flow and energy resources into our bodies and lives.

the connection to spirit in your female body allows you to access the infinite creative resources your spirit contains.

Whether you conceive a child, sustain a pregnancy, hold an energetic space for adopting or stepparenting a child, have a miscarriage, or give birth, there are openings in the field around your body that allow you to access and receive energy from the spiritual realm. I have had the profound experience of witnessing this capacity and even using it to help women heal from disruptions in these energy transfers or create new patterns of motherhood. *Mothering from Your Center* shares the tools for you to access this creative potential in your own body. To begin this process of aligning the pelvic bowl, I have found it helpful for women to explore three aspects of energy medicine I use in my women's health practice:

1. Clarifying your field

2. Engaging your creative blocks

3. Focusing your creative desires

Clarifying Your Field

Clarifying your field means learning to sense and align energy as a way to organize your energetic space. It is helpful to clarify your body's energy field as preparation for conception and birth events and to enhance the flow in everyday mothering. As you become aware of your own energy field and how much lighter it feels when it's clear, then you can also clarify the energy around your connection to your partner, the energy fields of your children, and the energy field of your home.

Energy is the essence of life that flows through and around us. When the energy field is clear, the energy flows more abundantly and fluidly, just like a free-flowing river. We can also have densities in the energy field, places of energetic or physical stagnation where the energy becomes sluggish and reduced.

Just like a neglected closet seems to attract clutter, the energy around us and where we live can become stagnant or cluttered unless we know how to clarify this space. It takes practice and sensitivity to be able to feel energy and the field that contains it, but everyone has the capacity to sense energy. If you have a child who is particularly sensitive, he or she likely already senses energy and benefits tremendously from having a parent who understands how to clarify and align the energy field.

Clarifying your field may include doing a specific meditation, receiving bodywork, taking a walk in the fresh air, or exercising. When you take care of your body and encourage your children to do the same, you increase the alignment of the body's energy field. If children are moody or if you or your partner are moody, moving the body will move the energy and often clear the stagnation that is otherwise blocking your inner flow.

Energy and the Home

The practice of feng shui, or placing objects in places that help align the flow of a room, is an example of energy medicine in practice. By caring for our home and organizing the physical space that nourishes us, we enhance the clarity of the energy field in the home and the people who live there.

Every time I reorganize the toys and play space, my children come along and begin to play with new vigor and inspiration. They are responding to the enhanced energy flow with a greater flow in their creativity. Notice how, when you clean your house or make special preparations for a party, your body feels good being in the well-tended space. In fact, tending your home helps organize the energy field around your body. When there is alignment in the home, the body responds to this energetic clarity and order.

Likewise, if you have been busy and unable to tend your home, you will find that clutter accumulates and your family may be more prone to conflict or moodiness. Rather than focus on the conflict, start organizing the house and invite them to help. The energy field will become clearer, lightening everyone's energy.

One of my favorite exercises for clarifying the energy field of the home and everyone in it is making a spiritual bath. This ritual is from traditional healer Rosita Arvigo and comes from the Maya tradition. A friend from India told me that her grandfather often went through the house, blessing the energy with a similar water bath. The spiritual bath is akin to holy water and is at the top of my list for realigning the energy flow.

I make a spiritual bath to add vibrance to our home, prepare for special events, and help any family member who is moody or off-kilter in some way. My children often assist me in making one. The water blessing clarifies and restores the pristine radiance that flows in each one of us when our energy is aligned.

Exercise: Making a Spiritual Bath

1. Fill a bowl with water. Gather some leaves or flowers, particularly from plants that you are drawn to—aromatic herbs and roses are ideal. As you gather the plant material, say a prayer, asking in your own way for divine assistance. One at a time, place a flower petal or leaf into the water. When you have finished gathering, notice the beauty created in this bowl.

2. Using your hands, squeeze the plant material into the water while saying a prayer. Ask for the healing, protection, or blessing that is needed. As Rosita, in passing on the teachings of Maya healer Don Elijio, says, "Trust—with all your heart—that blessings will come to you." Notice the quality of air or energy that surrounds you.

3. Leave the bowl outside for an hour or so to continue to receive the earth blessings that create a natural alignment of energy flow.

4. Return to the bowl and squeeze the plant matter once more with thanks and prayer. Place most of the plant matter on the ground. Then begin to clarify your own energy by splashing water into the air around your body, like a bird taking a bath.

Imagine the blessing of this water extending into your wild feminine landscape to brighten all the energy that comes into or radiates from your center.

5. Sprinkle the blessing water around the energy field of each family member (or invite them to splash themselves). Sprinkle the water around your home, clarifying the energy field of each doorway and room. Include your animal companions as well. When you have finished, pour this blessing water onto the earth, with gratitude.

Engaging Your Creative Blocks

Creative blocks are the recurrent densities in your energy field that limit alignment and flow, and they are the next focus of the energy work I recommend. Encountering energy blocks and resistance to creative flow can be challenging, but, when engaged, they become some of your best assets for restoring a more robust vitality. Restoring energy flow in these places of stagnation is the key to accessing hidden creative potential.

To engage with your creative blocks, let go of the stories and emotions that may be contributing to your resistance. Instead, seek them out at the simplest level by feeling the sensations in your body when they arise. Do you encounter a sense of creative blockage in regard to a specific aspect of mothering, a particular task in tending your home, your ability to access the passion in your life, or the cultivation of one of your creative dreams? When you find a specific block, explore it with your senses in full detail. What does it feel like? Is it soft or hard, thick or thin, heavy or brittle? The more curious you can be about the creative block sensations in your body, the better you can sense what is there; sensing the energy is essential to being able to work with and transform the restricted pattern that contains it. Rather than fixing your past, you are changing the energy imprint in your center. The next two sections contain specific examples of working with creative blockages.

Meeting the Mother Line

Many women worry about becoming a mother because of their own painful relationship with their mother or other difficulty from childhood. As a spiritual practice, mothering calls you to meet your mother line—the lineage of mothers that stands behind you—and fully take your own place there.

Working in the female pelvis, I have seen that unresolved mother-line issues affect the creative flow in every woman, whether she becomes a mother or not. Even our relationship with the term or concept of *mother* determines how we access or block our creative essence. The additional step of having a child—a step that initiates your official motherhood—simply makes these energetic patterns and densities more visible so that you can engage them directly.

If you had a difficult relationship with your mother, you may form an energetic blockage and avoid becoming a mother or resist your mothering role. Or whenever you think of or interact with your mother, you may feel patterns of tension in your body. You do not need to heal your mother to change these patterns.

Rather than trying to relax your body when you think of your relationship with your mother, notice the specific sensations within the tension pattern. By feeling the sensations of the resistance in your body and energy field, you can move the core restriction. It seems simple, and it is actually a simple process, yet most people focus on the cause of stress (in this example, the mother relationship) instead of bringing presence to the sensations it produces in their body. Though the relationship may still be difficult, working with and attending to the energy blockages in your own body gives you the most power to change the way you hold the energy for yourself. In fact, by becoming aware of the sensations within an energetic block, you may shift an imprinted pattern with little to no resistance.

We carry our lineage, from both our mother and father lines, at a cellular level. There are physical and energetic imprints of our ancestors in the body and ways of being. When women express worry about passing on limiting patterns to their children, I share that because of our intimate bodily connections, from in utero and even as an egg in the ovary, as well as the daily caretaking, we cannot help but pass along patterns to our children. With our presence and support, our children will also cultivate and transcend these patterns; they will take what they have been given and make their own patterns.

Fortunately, even in families with difficult or painful histories, our complex family energies may contain threads or energy lines that resonate and can be taken up and celebrated anew. Savor the beneficial lineage patterns—like a talent for gardening, math, humor, music, networking, or cooking. Review those that are limiting—like a lack of self-worth, inability to express oneself, shame regarding the body, or difficulty in connecting with others. It is by acknowledging the imprints that we can begin to change them, particularly by sensing how our bodies respond and then reengaging our full potential. Drawing strength from the beneficial patterns and evolving beyond the limitations, we can amend our inherited forms.

It is not essential to resolve a relationship with a particular parent or person to change your own lineage imprints. Rather, it is by clarifying your energy field and restoring the flow in places of stagnation that you bring a more robust quality to your creative center and mothering life. Giving to your children also heals you.

Take the opportunity that mothering presents to work with your lineage energy, and you will find undiscovered potential. The burdens of your line, once addressed, will liberate your creative flow. Chapter 8 shares additional tools for transforming a painful lineage in regard to mothering.

What are the gifts of your lineage?
What are the challenges of these lines?
How will you transform what you have been given?

Releasing My Vacuum Rage

I inherited a pattern of rage-filled housecleaning. Anger was frequently expressed in my house while I was growing up, and the intensity of anger increased markedly when the house was being cleaned. I later had a tremendous block to cleaning, particularly in regard to vacuuming my own house, especially once I had children.

Stepping into the role of mother brings to light more of your lineage issues. We all have patterns that we carry from our lineage. Some of them are beneficial and others are limiting. I have a love of children, my female body, and the feminine realms of birthing and being a mother. These are patterns I carry from my own mother, who loved these things as well. I have relied on these strengths in birthing my children, being a mother, tending a home, and even being able to cherish the female body as I do in my work. However, there are also challenges I have had to contend with. One is my own anger and the stress patterns that might activate it in toxic ways.

To be able to vacuum after encountering my housecleaning energy block and sense of internal rage that accompanies it, I had to stop myself repeatedly (while vacuuming) and notice the specific sensations I was feeling in my body. I felt tension, as if I were being squeezed, and a sense of overwhelming pressure. I recognized the pressure as a feeling that there was a tremendous burden of tasks to be done and no possibility for rest. Yet I knew that I could take breaks if I chose to; the intensity of my feelings did not match the actual situation. When an emotional weight is greater than the reality surrounding us, it may be an amplification of the past and our lineage patterns.

My mother and her mother both had intense workloads, including children and financial stresses, which took a tremendous toll. On the outside, they are quite different people. However, as mothers, they shared a similar devoted love for their children, combined with a sense of daily stress and pressure that rarely abated.

Taking breaks in the midst of my own vacuuming, I slowed down my inner response long enough to recognize the bodily imprints of this stress and pressure in myself. Each time the sensations of stress would build, I would stop and breathe to regain my center. By laying my body on the ground, I could release the energy to the earth and with it the sense of building stress. Rage tends to rise, and moving it instead toward the ground made a different route for the energy to release.

By interrupting my housecleaning to attend to my inner needs, I was reframing my embodied pattern of mothering to include rest and renewal. I was also retraining my nervous system to comprehend that stress did not mean full-steam-ahead work, ending only when I erupted in rage. By stopping, I also encountered vast layers of grief and my unmet needs and those of my mother line. I incorporated counseling and bodywork from gifted healers to clear these imprints from my field and make room for the life-enhancing flow of joy.

Vacuuming also creates an energetic charge, which my body is sensitive to. When the ground is warm, stepping outside and standing on the earth with bare feet can clear this charge (or even the charge from computers and electronics). Additionally, breathing the fresh air and drinking water is helpful. This charge effect is worse when I am menstruating, so I avoid vacuuming during this time. During menstruation, female energy systems are more open in order to assist our bodies in clearing energy, and they are more sensitive to external energies as well.

Energy blocks can also be engaged in a playful manner. When my first son was a toddler and enamored with costumes, I wore a pair of fairy wings while vacuuming one day. It is difficult to feel rage while wearing fairy wings. Switching from rage to playfulness, the densities in my center became lighter in response. Over time, the blocks softened. I sensed them with compassion, understanding the burdens that women carry. Now I vacuum with ease, bringing my cleaning fairy to the task of clarifying our home. Having healed this lineage imprint, my energy system is no longer held hostage by the rage pattern. I gained back an immense part of my creative range to use as it was intended—for creating more beauty in my life. Now I am working on my patterns around cooking.

What are your energy blocks in mothering?

What happens when you engage these blocks instead of avoiding or resisting them?

How can you access more of your wild feminine landscape, the creative capacity in your center?

Focusing Your Creative Desires

A woman who knows what she wants is a force of nature. By clarifying your energy field and engaging the blocks or lineage patterns that would limit your creativity, you can then shift your attention to the most essential aspect of your creative fire: what you want to create. We have a choice about what we hold in the center. Particularly once we free our creative essence from restrictive patterns, we can turn our focus toward the vast potential of this life force within.

As you tune in to your unique rhythms, your mothering essence will change over time. Your motherpiece is an evolving reflection of your creative inspiration. In becoming a mother, you may first step into a place of scarcity and wounding. With the emphasis of modern culture on achievement outside the home, you may feel forgotten or isolated in returning home to tend your child. As the feminine rises, however, more people will be called to tend their inner fires, whether in mothering or other ways. Take heart that the energy in the home will strengthen as the return to the home continues on many levels. In fact, many mothers also feel surprised by the sustenance they enjoy in tending the children and home. Contrary to the feminist movement, which necessarily freed women from their domestic lives, time has evolved, and more women—and men—are coming home.

Do your work now: Add to your motherpiece. Cultivate a vibrant home fire that nourishes you and your family. Seize the opportunity that motherhood brings for retreat, and contemplate your retreat as a creative rebirth for yourself. Every artist knows that retreating to the inner space is essential for meeting the creative muse. Ponder the essence of your own creative motherhood; envision and then manifest your radiant form.

TWO

Engaging the Mystery in Your Womb

On one of the last autumn nights after my mystical miscarriage, we built a fire under the stars. The darkening sky carried the first chill of fall. In the backyard, bordered by roses and raspberries, I felt held. The wood from our fire gave off a piney smoke. I wrapped my wool shawl around my shoulders. The flowers still lingered where we had laid the tiny being I had miscarried at the end of the summer.

Since the bright August day of my mystical journey, I had been tending the spirit door, this sacred place in the female body where a soul can enter—and leave from as well, I had learned. By tending to the grief that flowed through my womb, I had freed myself of so many burdens.

My own being felt light as I stood on the smooth brown earth. Like a gardener who has done the work in her garden, I was learning the way of these ancient creative cycles. The seasons were changing, and I was leaving the tender ground of this loss in care of the earth. There was a creative current moving through my body, and the end of one cycle marked the beginning of another.

Lifting my eyes from the fire, I saw my two-and-a-half-year-old son dancing in the shadows cast by the fire's light. He was weaving in and out of shadows and light, like a flame himself. My husband came near, and we watched the fire in silence. Each time we have encountered another of life's unexpected turns, I have been amazed by the beauty that eventually arises.

We lingered in the warmth of the fire, hesitant to leave such peace. I walked inside slowly, followed by my son. Filling a glass with water in the kitchen, I said, "That was lovely."

"What?" my son asked. "That spirit I was playing with?"

I turned to him. "What, honey?"

He repeated, "Mom, are you talking about the little boy spirit I was playing with?"

I bent down so that I could see his face. "You were playing with a spirit?"

He answered, "Yes, a little boy spirit. It was fun."

I pondered this gift from my son: *A little boy spirit*. After taking time to heal from the miscarriage, we had just begun to invite another baby into our lives. Perhaps I would be tending the spirit door again soon.

Energy Medicine for Conception and Pregnancy

Even as modern medicine has evolved, conception and pregnancy continue to remain a mystery. By working with the energy of the pelvic bowl, we can cultivate a relationship with this mystery. Though we cannot control our fertility, we can align ourselves with an inner creative flow and discover the potential of this elemental life force within. Working with the light of our own center, we can receive the flow of life coming into form, whether as a tangible creation or as lessons for being in the company of spirit.

I have developed a set of energy-medicine exercises that can help during general conception and pregnancy, as well as during fertility assistance. When conception and pregnancy come with effort, or not at all, the risk is to set oneself up to feel like a failure or, alternately, to try everything in the hopes of being "good enough" to conceive. Difficulty in achieving pregnancy can cause great pain in a woman's heart. I have witnessed the bountiful creative energy in women who are ripe with fertile essence yet cannot seem to conceive or hold a pregnancy; it is puzzling. I offer these exercises to assist your fertility journey, but even more than achieving a certain outcome, I hope that they will deepen your relationship to the mystery of your body. Aligning the energy of our bodies can support our fertility, but it is essential to love ourselves no matter how our journey with fertility unfolds.

The Inner Creative Potential

The first priority in preparing for conception is to make a connection with your pelvic bowl and womb. Since many women are delaying pregnancy and using birth control, they have often unconsciously conveyed an internal "no" to their womb regarding pregnancy. Ten or twenty years of fertile time may pass in which they have unintentionally but energetically repressed the creative potential of the body.

Ideally, we establish an intimate relationship with the womb and our internal creative nature before contemplating children— setting up an inner dialogue to cherish and use our creativity in designing a vibrant life. I teach women in my practice to cultivate a connection with the creative center because when we have not had children, whether or not we choose to have them, we can unintentionally close ourselves off from this inner potential. As modern women with more choices around fertility, we can still align our-selves with the creative womb and ovarian energy in all aspects of life—to feel our vibrancy, to make a career that fuels our passion, and to engage in dynamic relationships with others.

When a woman decides to have a child, there may be pent-up frustration in the womb. I know this to be true because I sit with women in these most intimate parts of the female body. Most mod-ern women embody a masculine pattern of *doing* and *driving* that goes counter to the more feminine, internal, and cyclical nature of the womb. For years, regardless of whether a woman is menstruat-ing or in a more restorative mode, she uses products and continues moving as if there were no inner cycle at all. Then, after the womb has been dragged along and ignored through relentless career devel-opment and other linear tasks, a woman may suddenly demand the womb's participation in having a baby. Does this sound familiar?

There is another way.

Reconnecting with the Pelvic Bowl

When you begin to connect with the internal realm of the pelvic bowl, many women initially find pent-up feelings of grief, sadness, shame, fear, or anger. These feelings are based on unmet needs that tend to accumulate with life habits or work structures that require an external focus, often causing you to ignore your own center. Held emotions may also be from past traumatic events, the imprints of your lineage, or the denial of the feminine that are embodied within each one of us. Near these emotional energies, there is also a potent life force; many women also find a dazzling inner radiance when they contact the energies of the creative center.

Clearing stagnant emotional energies from your core allows you to restore the flow of creative vitality meant for your life. Rather than containing stored emotional energies, the pelvic bowl is designed for gestating your life creations. Once you reconnect to your pelvic bowl and stay long enough to clarify your core, you will discover that there lies a profound vibrancy in your center. This creative essence contains the sacred potential to generate life.

If you are having difficulty conceiving, it is not a measure of your connection to this mystery—it is simply not that personal. Women can become pregnant whether they are connected with the internal creative potential or not. My own feeling is that the energies of the earth have been diminished, and since our female bodies reflect the energy of the earth, we also reflect the dissonance of living out of balance. Whether facing this through challenges with fertility or the diseases in our children and ourselves, coming back to balance in the center is vital.

Still, life goes on. The regeneration continues within and around us. The best hope we have for healing ourselves and re-centering our world is for women to remember the wisdom of their own body, honor this life-giving potential within, and follow the truly sustainable rhythm that arises from the womb. Making a connection with the womb offers guidance in regenerating life and harmonizing our energies for living.

Cultivating a Feminine Approach to Conception

Modern women have typically adopted a masculine form of *production* in developing their professional careers. This linear and task-oriented way of operating tends to make the energy more focused and targeted. Masculine energy is not gender specific, although males embody the masculine more readily. My young sons exhibited early on a need to externalize and project energy by hitting or throwing. Still, females can run on masculine energy as well. Many women in the business world have learned the masculine form of projecting energy in order to drive and lead a company.

The energy of the womb, and place of conception, carries the opposite and complementary energy to this linear and masculine movement. The womb is round, receptive, and feminine. It embodies the power of the feminine, which lies in being, or holding space, rather than *doing*. I encourage women to intentionally soften themselves to prepare for conception. The more soft, feminine, dreamy, and non-time-based they become, the better for cultivating the feminine aspects of their energy.

Measuring temperatures and checking ovulation is a task-oriented process that will increase your masculine essence. To aid conception, avoid the mental or linear focus as much as possible and instead dip into the mystery. Follow your body's desires and let yourself be open to the passion with your partner. If assessing ovulation is necessary, do it in a relaxed and fluid way. Make love spontaneously around the suggested timing as well, because true ovulation can occur outside an ovulation window. Your body may know better if you can restore your womb connection and tune in to your feminine intuition.

When you are making love, bring awareness to your vagina and your womb. Feel your partner from there and invite his essence, his penis, and his sperm to move deeply inside you. Open yourself like a flower to his penetrating masculine energy. This fusion of masculine and feminine in lovemaking nourishes each partner and generates a potency for the relationship that creates life. Though this masculine-feminine fusion is found all around us in nature, you may need to clear away layers of shame or protection to receive the beauty of your partner in this way. Remember the sacredness of your connection and allow your feminine to receive his masculine.

Conception for Lesbians

What if your partner is not a he? If two women are using assistance to conceive, then I invite them to bless the sperm and the man who provided it, honoring this male whose essence will be a profound part of their child.

Many female couples are able to inject the sperm in the privacy of their home or participate in the process in a clinic, so a similar energy dance unfolds. One woman is receiving the sperm and opening her feminine center to receive, and typically the other woman is using her essence in a more masculine way by helping to insert the sperm. Coming into a deep union and love for one another, regardless of gender combination, sets the conception field in a vibrant and life-giving way. One of the most important aspects of conception is finding resonance with your partner and creating a dynamic connection between you to conceive and then care for a child.

The following exercise can be done as preparation for conception or other creative ventures. It can also be practiced prior to and during in vitro fertilization or fertility processes to activate the energy potential even in a medicalized process.

Exercise: Preparing for Conception and Alchemy Unfolding

1. Bring your awareness to the deep center of your pelvic bowl. This is the energetic space of the womb. Remember, this is the sacred place where spirit enters the female body. Take a moment to sense the expansive beauty within your female body.

2. In your mind's eye, take a walk around your pelvic bowl. Imagine a broom that you can use to sweep and clarify the energy within and all around you. With each inhale, take in fresh energy. With each exhale, clear away any energy that is no longer needed.

3. Now breathe into your center and soften the womb space. Let the cells of your center expand in order to receive the light of spirit there. Feel the breath of life meeting your breath.

4. Call in the essence of your partner. Imagine the love you
   share and the ways you ignite the passion and life force in one
   another. Let your combined energy fields expand the space
   held for this child.

5. Set a few intentions. What are you wanting to create? The
   womb is a sacred altar where you can place your dream seeds.
   Ponder your intentions and then set them tenderly in your
   own center. Imagine them there as sparks of light, blossoms,
   prayers, a fertilized egg, or whatever image or words will represent these precious seeds. Then lisen to your womb.

6. Allow these dream seeds to take root in your womb. Soften
   your center, move with your partner, and let the alchemy
   unfold.

7. Invite the light of spirit to touch the seeds of your creations.
   See the radiance of spirit coming into your center, blessing
   these dream seeds, and shining through your whole field. Let
   spirit tend these seeds while you return to the tasks of your
   day. Carry this bright potential with you wherever you are.

Resolving Fertility Challenges and Past Womb Losses

When conception and pregnancy are elusive or difficult, additional
support and energy tools are helpful. Each one of these tools was
developed by working with women on their fertility. They were
created to support the connection between a woman and her body
during a time when it may be greatly challenged.

Bringing more awareness to the womb, whether as pregnancy
preparation, conception, or giving birth, can stir up past losses,

including miscarriage, abortion, or other trauma. The energy of loss or trauma can be addressed to ease the way.

Women's Stories: Reclaiming Her Center

Katrina was having difficulty conceiving. In sharing her women's health history, she spoke about the personal effects of an abortion she had had ten years prior. At that time, abortion was a clear choice for her. However, she felt it was traumatic for her body. She had bled for an extended period. She also mentioned feeling a longtime disconnection from her pelvis.

Pelvic disconnect is a common issue in my women's health practice. In addition to learning to live outside our centers by focusing on school and careers, many women experienced early imprints of shame. This may be related to harsh potty training, negative messaging about the body, parents' discomfort with their own sexuality, past abuse or trauma, and even menstruation, femininity, or gender. When I work with a woman, my goal is to restore her connection to the powerful and fertile creative space in her body. Wherever there is pain or disconnection, there is also potential for healing.

With this in mind, I began the internal pelvic work to support the healing in Katrina's center. The first thing I noted was that Katrina's pelvic muscles were tense and hyperengaged. This tension can inhibit the blood and hormone flow in the pelvic bowl and inhibit conception. Her uterine energy pattern was also in a state of sustained holding. When a woman wants to conceive, her womb needs to be supple, open, and receptive. A uterine holding pattern sends the signal that her womb is energetically full and unable to receive.

Modern women have chronic uterine holding patterns because we continue to be busy even when our inner cycle suggests we rest. We also tend to be overly sedentary, which further increases pelvic stagnation. Again, if we continuously send an internal "no" signal to the womb regarding fertility, we further add to the stagnation rather than engaging this creative potential.

Additionally, Katrina relayed her abortion experience as a place of trauma for her. Pelvic trauma can cause a holding pattern related to shock. When I work with a woman to restore the womb energy flow and resolve a bodily response to trauma, I begin by massaging her inner pelvic muscles and inviting her to breathe toward her womb. Women benefit tremendously from reviving the pelvic bowl so that, rather than carrying an imprint of trauma, a sense of health and vitality is restored in the body.

In Katrina, I felt a pattern of strain in her center, from the pelvic fascia up toward the womb. A strain pattern can result from a previous fall and impact to the pelvis or can be related to a trauma such as her abortion.

As I massaged the fascial tension pattern in Katrina's pelvis, tears flooded her eyes and cascaded down her cheeks. "Tears are always welcome here," I shared. When we experience trauma in life, we do not want to stop our processing at the traumatic event. Trauma causes an energy disconnection—often, at the time, a protective effect that is a matter of survival—but a person's muscle and mental memories can become frozen and stagnant without further work. With our energy tools, we can restore the lost connection and revive the flow of energy to transform the trauma response.

However a woman experiences womb loss, her womb may hold the energy. Reconnecting to her center, even pondering the essence of the soul who came to her, can bring comfort. In this quiet and honoring reflection, the womb can release the held energy. I have felt these womb releases from women's bodies, flowing down and out like a rush of heat. With that release, the womb can rest and restore herself in order to prepare for receiving new life.

After our session, Katrina had a brightness in her eyes. "I feel like a whole woman again," she marveled. "I didn't realize how much I had lost touch with." Though working in the pelvic bowl does not always solve fertility challenges, Katrina did conceive about six months later. She felt that reconnecting to the life-giving potential in her body assisted conception and restored a profound connection to herself that continued to serve her pregnancy and mothering.

What losses have you experienced as a woman?
How might you receive healing in the place of loss and further reclaim your creative range?

Conception after Miscarriage or Birth Loss

When you have already known loss, it can be difficult to trust your body or your ability to sustain a pregnancy and birth a baby. Working with a counselor who specializes in womb loss can be helpful and often necessary, but then you still have to restore a connection with your body and the place of loss.

Women's bodies seem to universally hold on to the essence of the soul lost in miscarriage or birth. I serve as an energetic midwife in these cases, coaxing the womb energy into alignment with a woman's present state of nonpregnancy and then restoring the energy flow in her body. During pregnancy, the womb is in a state of holding while gestating a baby. With womb loss, however, the womb must release the energy in order to restore balance in a woman's center, just as the physical release completed. This energetic release actually assists her connection with the soul of her child, because then the spirit connection flows through her rather than remaining tucked within her womb. (See the section on healing the womb from miscarriage and birth loss in chapter 5 to explore this topic further.)

Energy Medicine for Working with Fertility Specialists

Preparing the womb as a feminine and receptive place can be helpful in working with fertility specialists, but it can also be challenging, since you are often in a medical office where your body may feel tense and guarded. I recommend having a daily meditation practice at home so that when you enter the office you can bring a practiced skill for relaxing your body even in a stressful situation. If it is possible, play some music or repeat a specific meditation while you are in a relaxed state, to facilitate your ability to center yourself within a medical office. The body is a creature of habit. Practice with breathing, music, and visualization to cue your body and create a balanced energy field as assistance for any medical procedure.

Fill a spray bottle with some water from a spiritual bath (page 13) and spritz yourself in the medical office for energetic support. You may also say blessings for the staff involved in the process, the fertilized eggs, the room, and your own body; this will help create a vibrant conception field even in the midst of a medicalized process.

Opening to Spirit: Expansion Versus Limitation

Many women who undergo fertility treatment feel an immense pressure to conceive and sustain a pregnancy, and then a profound sense of loss and failure when the fertility attempts "fail." In the process, they often experience a growing sense of limitation and creative blockage.

It is essential for a woman to relieve the bodily tension caused by these fertility challenges. Massage and other relaxing body treatments can be helpful, as well as meditation practices that align her with an ever-present potential for creative energy. Feeling limited by her options or outcomes will contract the energy field; focusing on the potential opens her energy field to the greater realm of spirit.

Whenever we feel stress or a lack of abundance and support in our life, there is a tendency to close ourselves in protection, holding tension in the body and constricting our energy flow. If instead we open ourselves to spirit, connecting our energy to the pulse of life, we can access these expanded energy resources that extend beyond our own capacity and offer a fuller, more energetic protection. Maintaining a balanced energy field with full access to our creative resources, regardless of external circumstances, is a tremendous gift to ourselves.

Exercise: Opening to Spirit in the Body

1. *Bring awareness to your body.* Notice where you hold any sense of limitation in yourself. Feel how these perceived limitations cause contraction both physically and energetically in your center and block the energy flow.

2. *Think of something that conveys worry or scarcity.* Notice the increased contraction response in your body and the shift or stagnation in your energy. Ponder places of lack or creative challenge and observe your core energy pattern.

3. *Make a connection with these places of stagnation.* Rather than simply trying to be rid of your challenges or blocks, simply notice and connect with the sensations they produce in your body and energy flow.

4. *Now ponder a favorite place on the earth or something that makes you happy.* Sense your body and energy as you do so. Your body relaxes and your energy expands toward the greater potential around you. Remember the wild feminine landscape. When you feel the gifts of your life, you inhabit the outer ring of spirit potential.

5. *Invite the greater energy from spirit to fill your center.* Ask for blessings and receive this energy. Remember your own sacredness. This journey is not about doing the right thing or being perfect but about understanding your inherent perfection and alignment with the divine. Let yourself find resonance with this sacred life force that flows through you and everything. Let it hold you even when—or especially when—you are challenged.

6. *Allow yourself and your family to be held by spirit.* Let the divine hold any challenges, emotional pain, or energy blocks. Open your energy field to the sacred, regardless of the external circumstances; access to this eternal source of unconditional love is your birthright.

7. *Give thanks for your beauty.* Ask this inner light to illuminate your way.

Energy Medicine for Adoption and Stepparenting

When a woman adopts a child or mothers a stepchild, she can still hold energetic space in her womb for that child, even if her child is no longer an infant. In asking my clients who were adopted how they sense the energy of their birth and adoptive parents, they describe the birth parents as a layer right at the core and then the adoptive or stepparents as a broader layer around them. In societies where there is a more tribal approach to child-rearing, a child is held by many people and benefits from a community of caregivers.

If you are planning to adopt a child, establish a daily pelvic-energy meditation practice, such as the Preparing for Conception and Alchemy Unfolding exercise (page 27). Hold the potential for your child in the womb space, and when you have a specific referral, hold this child with intention. It is also helpful to use blessings: *May this child be blessed. I give thanks for his/her birth parents, and may they be well. Bless our family and bless the adoptive process.* Blessings align the energy field and facilitate the flow that will bring your child to you.

For any challenges you encounter in the adoption process or as a stepparent, bring a blessing instead of a worry, as this will align, rather than constrict, the energy. With adoption, there is the period of waiting for your child, which can be filled with either anxiety or anticipation. In stepparenting, there can be difficulties with ex-partners or resistance from the children you are responsible for. By using the energy tools to clarify your center and bless yourself as a mother, you can ease the various connections and lighten your experience of mothering even in the midst of challenges.

In preparing to be a mother by adoption or as a stepparent, it is helpful to establish a relationship with your own creative essence, especially if you have had fertility issues. Sometimes women carry a sense of failure or shame in their center in regard to their fertility, or they may feel unsure about how to engage their mothering center in relation to a child born to someone else. Likewise, consciously connecting to your creative center establishes the connection and flow that is normally stimulated by giving birth. Know that your womb space is essential for mothering and connecting with every child you hold dear.

Read each of the exercises in this book with the potential of children held by your energy connection, no matter how they come to you. In chapter 7, you'll find additional resources to access the energy of your center for mothering or stepparenting a child of any age.

Pregnancy Energy by Trimester

Pregnancy alternates between pure delight at the miracle within and the more pedestrian tasks of choosing a care provider, deciding on in-utero testing, and preparing for labor. You will be transformed by the child unfolding in your center. Sometimes it means moving your entire living space or initiating other significant changes in your life. Even as you consider making decisions for your pregnancy, listen to your own center and draw upon the ancient wisdom that resides there to engage the mystery at each step.

The First Trimester: A Star Unfolding

With each pregnancy, I experienced a moment where I felt a tingling in my center, as if a tiny cosmos were unfolding. In fact, it is. The fertilized egg travels to the womb and finds a place to land. The womb cradles the precious new life, and the star inside expands and unfolds, drawing in and upon the potent life-force energy.

Though the medical establishment would have women go about their business during the first trimester—just like we are encouraged to keep our same pace even while menstruating—I disagree. The first trimester is a delicate time. The cells are fragile and the bond between the early hint of baby and womb is still tenuous.

It is wise to rest, shelter yourself, and let life take hold. Similar to preparing for the arrival of winter, slow your pace from running to walking. Read books, make fires, eat well, and rest. Nausea also serves to slow us down. Unless it is summer, keep your pelvis and womb covered with layers for warmth. Stay hydrated and avoid air travel if you are able, as flying is quite stressful to the body (and baby). If you have to fly, stay well hydrated.

Let yourself enter the dreamy state that pregnancy invites. Pregnancy represents a nine-month journey to the birth point, and there is a corresponding nine-month journey to the other side, during which you leave the linear and logical world behind. For some, this is upsetting because their lives are rooted in a linear construct that corresponds to being organized and structured. For others, they are happy to leave behind the boxes that were too limiting anyway. Either way, shed the old and embrace what comes; let yourself be moved and changed.

The first trimester carries a hint of the sweetness coming to you, but it can also make you feel unmoored. When we go through any major transition, there is a natural vulnerability in the process of shedding our former structures, identities, and energy patterns. We also feel more vulnerable because our energy fields are more open to receiving the incoming energy of pregnancy and a new being, sensitizing us to everything.

Because many miscarriages occur during this time, early pregnancy can feel tenuous in other ways. A woman may hesitate to bond with the baby in her center until she is assured that he or she will stay. However, faith requires opening to what is—without knowing the outcome. Let yourself receive the blessing in your center. In chapter 5, you will find energy medicine for miscarriage and birth loss. Though loss is undesired and difficult to comprehend, tending to a womb or birth loss can invite a profound connection to spirit.

After my own miscarriage, I was more aware of the link from spirit to womb. One day, early in my pregnancy with my second son, I was particularly nauseous and kept trudging along through various tasks. Finally, I had mercy on myself and lay upon the couch. As soon as I stopped my activity and focused on my womb, the nausea lightened—the beauty of rest and the art of being. I was building my baby's body and bringing in the essence of a new soul. Remembering this, I concentrated on softening my center and making my cells as open as possible to receive the energy for this child.

Upon closing my eyes, my feeling sense perked up. I felt a broad ray of warmth coming from a faraway place in the sky and toward my belly, like light from a distant star. *I wonder if this is his energy.* I let the warmth come into my center, and the nausea dissipated. Perhaps the energy was traveling a long distance, and my body was having difficulty integrating it until I consciously opened my energy field.

I lay on my soft brown couch, pondering the mystery of the stars, pondering the mystery of the star unfolding in my center.

The Second Trimester: Taking Root

In the second trimester, the baby and womb have made a more secure connection. The pregnancy is taking root, and the mother may feel strong and energized by her growing belly. Fears may arise or, alternately, life may seem bright with potential as the pregnancy unfolds, each one uniquely.

This is the period to savor the pregnancy experience. Join a community of pregnant women, whether by taking prenatal yoga, prenatal water aerobics, or a birth class. Prepare the baby's room and read books about birth and parenting. One of my favorite birthing books is *Spiritual Midwifery*, by renowned midwife Ina May Gaskin. It is filled with women's birth stories written in their own words. The book is from the 1970s, and the "birth is psychedelic" language reflects the era, but the stories gave me a bodily imprint of birth before I had my own initial birthing experience. They are empowering and helpful, setting up the energetic frequency of birth as natural and beautiful.

SUPPORTING OPTIMAL BABY POSITIONS FOR BIRTHING

Getting in shape physically will assist your body in birthing. In the second trimester, you may have more capacity to do so. However, be careful about vigorous exercise, as your pregnant body is less able to discharge heat and the fetus is vulnerable to high body temperatures.

Yoga is beneficial for relaxation, core strength, and overall flexibility but should be modified during pregnancy and nursing, as hormones cause laxity in joints and connective tissues, making ligaments prone to overstretching. This laxity helps your body accommodate a growing pregnancy and ease the birthing process, but care should be taken to avoid injury. Water aerobics allows you to exercise with the support of water, and the water also dissipates excess body heat. Walking helps increase overall health and vigor.

It is important to avoid sitting for long periods and to rest by lying on your side rather than leaning back on the couch. Babies tend to find a better position in the pelvis, particularly toward the end of the pregnancy, when a mother is moving or in an upright posture. Before our largely sedentary lifestyle, women were generally up and moving, rather than sitting, and it may be that the body incorporates this into the birthing process.

Extended sitting increases pelvic congestion, while body movement increases cellular flow and pelvic health. Sitting back tilts the pelvis and potentially shifts the baby into a posterior position, rather than the optimal anterior position, which aligns the baby's head and body to move more easily through the mother's pelvis while birthing. In the birth of my second son, a posterior position—where the back of baby's head is toward the back of the pelvis, often pushing against the sacrum—made for a more difficult and prolonged birth. If a woman or baby becomes too fatigued in prolonged labor, intervention can be a necessary support.

I wish that all women could hear as many stories of birth as I do, so they would realize that needing or accepting support in a difficult birth is not a sign of failure or weakness. No matter how much you prepare, every birth event is a unique set of circumstances, and an excessively long labor is not good for mom or baby.

Optimal baby positioning can make the difference between straightforward and difficult labor, and ought to be part of the pregnancy and birth education. The website SpinningBabies.com promotes "easier childbirth with fetal positioning." This site has a wealth of information regarding how to facilitate optimal birthing positions, including how to work with a baby in breech position. These techniques worked for me, and I have seen them work for others. With my third pregnancy, I was careful to sit upright and forward on my pelvis, to stay active, or to rest by lying on my side to help prevent a posterior position. My third birth event was more rapid, with a straightforward progress through the birth canal, partially due to my baby's optimal position.

The Third Trimester: Moving toward the Spirit Door
As a woman enters the third trimester, she is moving closer toward the spirit door. This is the time for her to prune away excess commitments and clear a wide space on her schedule in order to feel unpressured and fully able to enjoy the birth and postpartum period.

In my first prenatal yoga class, we had a ritual in which the mothers who had given birth returned to share their birth stories. Hearing these stories prepared those of us still pregnant in making our own way to the spirit door. One woman shared her realization that going toward the labor pain was the way to open her body and womb for birthing, rather than simply avoiding it or trying to be comfortable. That struck me as I realized I had been thinking that the goal of laboring was to find positions of comfort. Yet labor "pain" or the intensity of labor is different from any other sensation; it is part of the expansion process that allows the body to birth a baby.

I would describe these sensations of birthing as an exquisite opening in the center of one's being. I prepared for my labors like spiritual quests, where my essence expanded multidimensionally and the intensity of the process opened a broader channel of creative flow and purified the cells of my being. Rather than travel to a remote spiritual destination, I saw this path as a holy trek through the body to retrieve the sacred essence of mother and child.

In preparing for your own labor, seek out stories of women who have been there. Stories engage a more holistic and less linear aspect of ourselves that is helpful for birthing. The book *Birthing from Within*, by Pam England, also offers creative exercises designed to engage the body's senses and prepare for birthing by going beyond our mental processes. Birth can even be pleasurable. Be inspired by the video clips of women savoring the sensations of birth in Debra Pascali-Bonaro's film *Orgasmic Birth*. Prepare for birthing by making daily pleasure a priority.

Pregnancy and birth are bodily events, rooted in the core of the body. The more you can connect to your body and the physical and energetic expansion that is unfolding, the better prepared you are to access the resources there. By the third trimester, there can be discomfort and a sense that pregnancy will never end. Staying with the sensations of discomfort and even finding your way to pleasure will enhance your ability to do so in labor. The exquisite expansion necessary for birth is assisted by moving toward, rather than away from, its intensity.

I have come to understand the spirit door as an opening in the energetic field. The birth is not only of the baby's body but also of this soul's life essence and the energetic information to provide mothering and care. It is a sacred process akin to the soul journeys of shamans. Because modern culture lives largely separate from the natural rhythms of the earth, we have mostly forgotten the spiritual and energetic aspects of birth as well as death. These life and death processes are related: the energy moves in for life, with our first inhale, or moves out in death, with our last breath. Waking up to the energy potential in our bodies as women, we can assist the culture in remembering the truth of our entry as spirit embodied. Remembering this truth, we will be better equipped to make a life that is soul-based and connected to our full creative potential, as well as to die with more peace.

The first time I went to the spirit door to give birth, I felt a rush of excitement to meet my child and recalibrate my life. More than a decade later, having been there several times now in birth and miscarriage, and working on the alignment of the spirit door with women, I know that this is truly a divine process. As women, our bodies directly download the sacred information for each soul and the soul of our communities. Prepare to witness nothing less than this in your own journey there.

The Art of Presence in Pregnancy (and Beyond)

One of mothering's greatest gifts is that it invites you to be in the moment, which increases your presence in the center of your life and your being. Bringing presence or expanded awareness to your center can allow you to savor your pregnancy or your child, but it can also bring you in contact with fears and other uncomfortable emotions.

I hear women voice fear about topics like becoming a mother, giving birth, the pain of labor, experiencing change, changes in the body, changes in their partnership, having a difficult birth, the health of their child, their own childhood wounds, safety and loss, miscarriage, losing their identity, balancing work and home, gender issues, being able to bond, being a good mother, and so on. Given the amount of transformation that mothering calls us to, these fears are relevant. However, fear is constrictive and limits us, particularly when it remains buried. By allowing your fears and other emotions to arise, you can begin to release the emotional energy that otherwise blocks your creative flow. By talking with a friend or counselor, sharing what is happening with your partner, journaling, or even just acknowledging how you feel, you invite a movement toward the healing support and sense of restored power.

Seeking the Truth within Fear

Initially I was afraid to have a daughter. I became aware of my fear regarding daughters while pregnant with my first son. Given that I enjoy being a woman and working with so many women, I was curious and sought the truth in my gender-based fear.

I surmised that the fear arose from my wounds regarding the feminine. Somehow I thought that not having a girl would prevent me from delving into this painful region. However, I soon discovered that to preserve the feminine for my sons, I would still need to traverse this lost ground. Giving birth to a particular gender would not save me from addressing the early wounds in myself if I wanted to mother from a more whole place.

Upon the arrival of my third son, I felt both the blessing of three boys as a brotherhood and also the new fear that I might be overwhelmed by my male-dominated household. Raising my sons, I have found the truth in this fear. In the raucous household of wrestling and pure physicality that males bring, I can feel overwhelmed. Therefore, I am honest with my sons and ask them to work with me and calm themselves when their high intensity becomes too much for our small house. I also regularly savor their boisterousness, which infuses my life with tremendous joy and balances my highly feminine work.

Breaking down fear into something tangible and manageable requires that we assess the limitations and truths present in the fear. Negative feelings regarding a particular gender can arise from fear about our ability to raise either a daughter or a son. Our own insecurities can manifest as fears about who our children might become. There can also be fear that we will lack for something if we do not have the chance to raise a certain gender. It is helpful to acknowledge the fear and then assess what is actually true.

It is natural for fear to arise as we move closer to the spirit door. The movement of energy in your center that occurs in pregnancy and birth will bring to light areas of stagnation and congestion. As your energy field opens to receive your child's energy, giving attention to these congested areas offers you an opportunity to clarify energetic patterns that no longer serve you. Seen in this manner, fear and other blocks can invite discovery rather than contraction and withdrawal. In my personal and professional practice, I have observed that the best antidote for any fear or other rising emotion is facing it with presence and even curiosity. Making a practice of meeting your emotional energies in pregnancy also increases your capacity to learn from the challenges encountered in birthing and mothering your children.

> What fears are you encountering in pregnancy, birth, and mothering?
>
> What is the truth present in each fear, and how might you address it?
>
> How does your energy change when you engage your fear or other feelings that arise?

Exercise: The Power of Presence in the Center

Engaging emotional energy with the power of your presence is a practice. At any point in your mothering journey, this practice can be used to drop away from fear or other challenges and into the power of your center. With presence in your center, you can always call in energetic support as needed. Sometimes all that is required is to just be with what is. Use the following exercise to assist you.

1. Sense into your fear or any other difficult emotion or situation. Notice how focusing on the limitation contracts and alters your energy flow or causes tension in the body. Do not judge your reaction; simply notice what happens.

2. Now bring your attention to the center of your pelvic bowl, to the womb space where you can connect with the peace and greater resources of spirit. Find the quiet, still place within, like an inner retreat. Often we attempt to fix or change what is happening; instead, be with what is. Expand your awareness into the space around you and simply notice the quality of your energy.

3. Ask this inner quiet place what you need or would like (rather than what is lacking or causing stress). Remember the power of your creative center, and say to yourself, *I would like* ... and state your desire as specifically as possible.

4. Envision an image of what it looks and feels like when this creative desire is fully realized. Energize this vision by witnessing it with your full presence, making energetic space for it to exist. Set your focus on this potential.

5. Offer thanks to your creative center. Bring this potency into the rest of your day or to any challenge that may arise.

Navigating Prenatal Tests and Ultrasounds

Whether or not to undergo prenatal testing is a personal choice for each couple. Some women may want every piece of data that is available during the pregnancy process; for other women, the plethora of prenatal tests can diminish the sense of sacredness and cause undue fear. It is important to take the time to tune in and feel what is right for you. Just as in raising a child, there are many ways to follow your inner guidance regarding care for your pregnancy and birth.

During my first pregnancy, a routine blood test returned a false positive for a serious genetic disorder, the screening for which I had not even realized was part of the lab panel. My whole body tightened in response. We elected to have an amniocentesis. I felt disconnected from my body until more than a week later we found that our baby was fine and healthy. Receiving the good news over the phone, I began to cry with relief. Simultaneously, my baby began to kick with sudden vigor, and I realized how my internal stress had affected him.

Interestingly, a few years later when I explained to my then three-year-old son the process of going to the hospital for birthing his baby brother, he became alarmed. He said, "You can't go there. They will try to stick him while he is in your belly." I looked into his frightened eyes. Was he referring to the amniocentesis I had had with him years before?

During the amnio procedure, we had watched our baby's movements as the doctor worked carefully to avoid touching him with the needle. I took the opportunity now to explain to him the amnio and its intention.

"You shouldn't do that, Mom. Babies don't like that," he said with a serious tone.

I hugged him. "I'm so sorry if it scared you. I wish I had been more aware of what babies feel. I only learned that after having you. Thank you for telling me." Acknowledging our children for all that they teach us can bring resolution.

I thought back to the amnio from my son's perspective. Though the doctor did not appear to touch my son's body in the procedure, even the puncture into the womb space may have felt like a violation. I imagine that babies in the womb have a more energetic sense of themselves, rather than having the defined boundaries of their bodies that comes with development. After the birth of my second son, I was holding him in my arms as we went in the yard to bury his placenta. My husband was placing the placenta into the earth when it slipped through his hands and landed with a soundless thud. In response, my son, who was just days old, startled in my arms as if he had felt the impact.

The Association for Prenatal and Perinatal Psychology and Health has published fascinating accounts and evidence regarding the imprinting that can occur in the womb, at birth, and as a baby. Though it is sometimes humbling to recognize the power of early imprints, mothering invites a direct relationship with this mystery of our coming into being. Our womb also contains energy medicine for healing the imprints that are less than ideal.

What plans do you have for supporting your pregnancy or birth or beyond?

How would you like to experience pregnancy, birth, or your body as sacred?

How is your mothering journey deepening your presence or connection to the mystery?

Practicing Presence in Pregnancy

Each time a woman becomes pregnant, she will encounter the energy that arises in preparation for this particular journey to the spirit door. Tapping into this energetic current, she can find guidance and inspiration for her creative and family life, or places to realign the energy.

To access the energy current coming in through the spirit door, pay attention to the themes that signal an expression of this new soul. There can be energy potentials and possibilities, opportunities for healing, places of growth, and clues regarding your shared life lessons. These energy currents accompany a baby's entry but can also be accessed by the whole family as part of the rich tapestry of living together.

What themes are arising during this or previous pregnancies?

What energy is coming in as you approach the spirit door in this or a previous birth?

How is the mystery in your womb unfolding at this time?

With my first son, I marveled at the physical strength that arose in my center during his pregnancy. I hiked, did yoga and water aerobics, and experienced a robust essence throughout carrying and birthing him. He continues to exhibit an incredible strength and physical prowess that defines many aspects of his life and brings abundant energy to our family. This physical thread that he brought in with him infuses his soccer playing, skateboarding, biking, paddle boarding, and so on. He introduces our family to new activities and catalyzes many adventures.

In birthing and mothering my second son, I had repeatedly learned about the connection between spirit and body and how tapping into this interface expands our creative potential. In my postpartum time with him, I envisioned a way to be with my family and expand my work from the home. Two years later, when my sons were two and five, we acted upon this vision to create a sacred space in our home with a wood-burning stove. This would be a place to retreat as a family, to make ritual, and for me to teach workshops. My second son has invited many occasions for sensing into the subtle layers of creative potential; he brings an expanded sensitivity and awareness into our family field.

By the arrival of my third baby, I had developed skills, from my years of mothering and working with women, for savoring the blessings of the present moment. Still, I had to examine an unexpected sense of fear that arose during his pregnancy. I was particularly worried as I approached his birth time, which seemed out of context because I was an experienced birther. It could have had something to do with switching to a home birth, but it felt deeper than that to me.

Sensing into the emotions with a trusted healer, I found that my fear was related to an experience from my father's childhood. When my father was three years old, and the youngest of three sons, he had a baby brother who was stillborn. Looking back as an adult, he remembered his desire as a child to comfort his mother by saying, "I'll be your baby." But it must have also caused a sense of profound loss and unease for him as well.

I lit a candle for my father's younger brother. I asked for a blessing on this baby, for my grandmother, and for my father, to soothe this early loss that was also carried cellularly within me. Perhaps it was the fact that I was birthing a third son that brought this layer to the surface. Either way, it was an opportunity to heal. Clarifying the energy field prior to my son's birth, by meeting and releasing these held emotions, I felt more space for celebrating his entry. Realigning with this river of energy that flows from the spirit door makes room to receive the blessings that each soul brings.

THREE

Birth: A Sacred Entry

B irth is an initiation, a passage through the gateway that brings your child into life and you into your mothering role. Your body expands to accommodate this new being and then gives birth to both the child's body and life force. Birth itself is an act of trust, and no matter how much you prepare, you will ultimately learn as you go. Still, preparations are necessary and can enhance confidence, ease fears, and otherwise help you feel more ready for labor and meeting your baby.

Tending to Birth Event Details

The birth itself requires the feminine ability to open and receive the energy of birth. Prior to the birth, however, the more masculine task-oriented nature can facilitate planning and organizing the

birth-event logistics. This type of planning is not intended to control the flow of the birth but rather to create a dynamic structure
that will support it.

Making a Birth Team

Finding a team of care providers who will best support your pregnancy and birth is essential. Some women make this selection based
on the connection they feel with a practitioner. While personal
chemistry is important, it is also essential to ask detailed questions
about the techniques used in birthing, what tests are performed
during pregnancy and whether they are optional, the transportation
plan if you intend to birth at home, how baby care is done
routinely after birth (such as placing the baby directly onto mom's
chest before washing—babies do not need to be washed right away
and mother's smell assists bonding), and what also occurs if your
baby should require some medical assistance.

In planning your birth experience, select a birth team and loca-
tion that align with your values and intentions for the birthing
process, including the monitoring and birth support techniques.
There are also different ways to monitor during labor, some less
obtrusive than others. Practices may range from not checking a
woman at all to checking her frequently, and it is important to consider what will feel best to you. Some women may feel reassured by
having birth providers check their labor progress, while others may
feel it interrupts their birth flow. I have also had clients whose birth
team was so hands-off during labor (whether at home or a hospital)
that the mother felt isolated or unsupported during the process.

With hospital births, practices vary from hospital to hospital, so
it can be helpful to talk to other women who have birthed at the
facility to find out about their birthing and aftercare experiences.
Will the staff read your birth plan? Does the hospital allow for
birthing and staying postpartum in the same room to reduce transi-

tions and increase the sense of family privacy? Do they offer water birth? Is the hospital oriented toward family needs and supportive of natural birth? Dr. Sarah Buckley's book *Gentle Birth, Gentle Mothering* is an insightful guide for making informed birthing choices, written from her broad perspectives as a physician and mother of four children. In fact, Dr. Buckley's findings about the physiological benefits of a natural and uninterrupted birth process influenced her decision to birth all her children at home with an emphasis on privacy, safety, and lack of disturbance during labor and birth.

If you are planning a home birth, ask about the type of support offered at home, how the birth team makes the call to transport you to the hospital if needed, and ways the birth team can support a hospital birth experience, including cesarean. I hear many women's birth stories, and advance knowledge is power. In my own planning for the home birth of my third child, I chose a birth team with a direct connection to a doctor at a hospital, to facilitate any transition that might occur. I asked more questions about baby resuscitation to ensure that my midwives had adequate skills. I also chose a team that would be more hands-on than hands-off. Because birth monitoring is already less a part of the home birth than a hospital birth, I did want some monitoring, as unobtrusively as possible, to ensure that the baby was tolerating labor well. I also wanted support if I needed it.

Once in labor, it is difficult to advocate for yourself. Ask the mothers in your community about their experiences and recommendations ahead of time. Keep in mind that your own intentions and energies will greatly influence your birth process; do your best to let go of the stories that do not resonate with you, such as worrisome labor experiences. Harvest the comforting details and release the rest.

Birth is a natural but quite intense process. Every woman has different needs in birthing, and every birth has its own process. The opening in the birth field and the birth energy flow have tremendous impact; taking time to prepare your support team is essential.

Setting Up the Birth Space

As you learn about birth, whether through books, videos, or birth classes, there is power in imagining what you desire for your own birth space. Consider whether you would like to birth on a bed or in a water tub, recognizing that every birth event has its own energy that may change or influence your actual choices during the birth. It is also helpful to have a doula (labor assistant) who has been at many births to assist your planning. This is particularly true if you will not have a midwife present. Most obstetricians are trained in surgery rather than labor, so you may choose to have someone at the birth who is experienced or trained in supporting a laboring woman.

Make a birth plan with any special requests such as birth position preferences, a dark or quiet birth room, delayed cutting of the placental cord, plans for the placenta (or a lotus birth, where the placenta remains in place until it naturally separates at the umbilicus), immediate breastfeeding, perineal care, and minimal intervention after the birth. Select music or special items for an altar. Gather baby things and wash the baby's clothes. Each step of preparation moves you closer to meeting your baby.

Remember to be flexible even as you try to plan. For example, for a first-time mother, the primary preparation for breastfeeding is to read about the skill. (Find more information about breastfeeding on page 92.) But the only way to learn how to breastfeed is by actually doing it. Having milk come in, obtaining a proper latch, working with the milk flow, and establishing a mother-baby nursing relationship are all affected by how things happen naturally. For example, sometimes a woman's breasts will produce milk with ease, while other times the supply is low. Or a woman encounters other challenges, like difficulty in the baby's latch. Each experience in birth and mothering calls for a dynamic response to meet each situation as it occurs.

The Blessing Way:
Celebrating New Patterns and Potential

Bringing presence to this sacred journey is work, but it is also an opportunity to celebrate the arrival of new patterns and potential. One of my favorite rituals for celebrating a pregnancy and cultivating helpful energies prior to birth is called a blessing way. Blessing way ceremonies can be varied in an endless number of ways, but the concept is to honor the mother and baby with a ritual. Friends gather to bless the mother and offer support with her transition into motherhood. They join with her to welcome the child approaching the spirit door.

In some ceremonies, friends will wash the new mother's feet in water scented with herbs. She might be massaged or anointed with oils. Some groups share readings or sing together as they tend to her. In some, participants are invited to call on the energies of the strong women in their lineage and lives.

A blessing way ritual invites a creative process or movement. One option is the creation of a birth necklace, made from beads gathered by the group. It can be worn by the pregnant mother or placed on an altar during the birth. It symbolizes the alignment and support gathered on behalf of the child and assists mother and child on their journey to meet one another. The necklace is typically too large to be worn by a baby, but it can be a treasured play item as the child grows and understands its meaning.

In my sons' birth necklaces, I was intrigued by how the beads often had certain themes, like wooden beads or glass or a certain type of stone, even though the gatherers did not consult together. It was as if there was a common essence that people responded to in choosing the beads. Like the energy of the spirit door and the child coming in was already making itself known. I have often sat with my sons, touching the beads with them and sharing the stories of our gathering while they were still in my belly. Their eyes brighten whenever we talk about this thoughtful ritual and creation made on their behalf.

Exercise: Making a Birth Necklace

1. *Preparation*: Invite friends to bring a few beads they are drawn to in anticipating your baby. Go to a bead store and purchase metal cord (thin enough for beads but strong enough to last). The bead store can help you clamp one end with a type of closure so the beads can be strung up to this closure point. Also select some smaller spacer beads that will be strung throughout the necklace.

2. *Opening*: Form a circle and open the ritual with a reading of a poem or blessing.

3. *Ritual*: Begin with some spacer beads, and then go around the circle and invite participants to place the beads onto the metal cord while sharing what inspired their choice. After placing their chosen beads, they can add some spacer beads and pass the necklace to the next person. Continue this process until the necklace travels the full circle. You can use a simple clamp to close the other end of the necklace yourself or temporarily secure it with tape until you return to the bead store. Another option is to pass around a bowl to collect the beads, which can be strung later. Some friends may offer stories about the reason they chose the bead, or about their connection to you.

4. *Setting intentions*: State your desires and intentions for this baby, the birth, and your family. Ask your friends to invite strong feminine energy from their lives, calling on mothers, grandmothers, sisters, and friends. They may also call upon

grandfathers, fathers, brothers, or others who have nourished and protected the family. It is vital to include men in our circle of awareness for honoring the sacredness of mother-hood. Invite these energies to join with you in weaving a strong support around this new or renewed family.

5. *Closing*: Close the circle with another poem or blessing. One of my favorite closings is a circle blessing: Gather hands and have each person say a blessing word, moving around the cir-cle. Travel the circle three times and savor the vibration of your collective blessing.

6. *Celebration*: Share a potluck meal, hot tea, or tasty dessert together, as you are so inspired.

Rearranging the Old Ways to Make Way for the New

A blessing way begins to align the energies around the mother as preparation and support for the energetic and physical components of birthing a child. It also provides assistance when she encounters the inevitable changes that lead to challenges along the way. In meeting these challenges myself, I have learned that rather than striving for a certain outcome, it is more helpful to invite spirit to assist the whole process of integrating new patterns and potential. And that rather than circumstances or events being particularly "good" or "bad," they are just the substance of living.

When we made my third baby's birth necklace, my oldest son was seven years old. Though he had cherished his own birth neck-lace for many years, he was envious of the new and shiny one made for our baby. My son and I talked about how the necklace creations were unique, created solely with one of them in mind. I thought our talk had settled him, until I found him hitting his birth necklace against a set of stairs. I came upon him right at the moment that his necklace shattered apart.

Having carried his birth necklace as a sacred part of his birth, and watching him carefully hold and play with it over the many years, I felt as if a family heirloom had been destroyed. I was shocked, but the horrified look on his face kept me from saying anything that conveyed my own emotions. In his expression, I read both the intent on some level to break it as well as his regret at actually having done so.

Together we began to gather the beads. "Wow, honey, your necklace . . . ," was all I could say.

"Do you think we'll find all the beads?" he asked worriedly.

"I'm sure. They're all in this one area. Let's just work together."

For the next thirty minutes, we searched the region around the wooden stairs to our basement. We were just a few feet from where we had created his brother's necklace and where his brother would later be born.

We placed all the beads from his necklace into a bowl. "I want to string it back together myself, Mom." And so he did. I gave him a metal string and clamped one end. He re-created the necklace. The beads had a new order, but they were arranged beautifully. Perhaps this was symbolic of his ownership of his birth energy. For me, it was a lesson in letting go of expectations and embracing the potential of what comes. Birth energy is powerful for the mother and baby but also for anyone in the family. Everything shifts when a new soul enters, and there is always some rearranging of the old patterns to make way for the new ones.

Touching the Spirit Door

It started at about eleven o'clock at night—strong contractions that signaled the beginning of labor with my second son. By one o'clock in the morning, the contractions were coming in regular waves through my body. My husband and toddler were sound asleep.

Pondering the rhythm of this second birth, I lay awake, watching my three-year-old sleep. Our world, and his world, were about to change. Another adventure into the unknown. A memory from the previous winter flashed to mind. I had been driving my son to a holiday party when, out of the blue, he said, "My brother is coming. It's been so long since I've seen him. I will be so glad to see him."

Struck by the clarity of his words, I asked him to continue.

"That's all, Mama," he said in his little voice. It was early December and I did not yet know that I was pregnant. Two weeks later, I would have a positive pregnancy test and, just before the new year, the nausea to confirm that another baby was on the way.

For the birth, we would again be at a local hospital. We chose this particular hospital for our first son's birth when I was working there as a physical therapist. I enjoyed my job, working full-time through my first pregnancy, and my husband felt more secure with a hospital delivery. Operated by the Sisters of Providence, the hospital has a rich practice of service. Every morning, an elderly nun recites a prayer over the intercom. I have an affinity for prayers from any tradition. While some hospitals have a coldness to them, this hospital attracts caring people who are aligned with a mission of service. I was comfortable there in the spacious birthing room with our beloved midwife, Karen, who would become a dear family friend.

Throughout the night, the contractions grew stronger and more regular. At four o'clock in the morning, I woke my husband. Should we take our son to the hospital with us? *Never wake a sleeping child* was one of my mantras. I knew my son would be confused and likely irritated by being pulled from bed in the middle of the night. I wanted him to be as rested as possible, to ease the coming transition. Already I sensed that this labor would be longer than the first one. We decided that my husband would stay home until daylight. I would go to the hospital and settle in.

Finding the Birth Flow

Every birth is exquisitely different. For my first son's birth, we arrived at the hospital with several bags, freshly brewed herbs as a perineal compress, and even a Crock-Pot to brew more herbs. I laugh now at how few of these things we actually used, but they added comfort to my first birthing experience. For this second birth, I just carried a small backpack with a few CDs, salt, herbs, sacred stones, and my baby's birth necklace—all to make an altar. Though my husband would later bring a larger bag with clothes for the baby and me, the items in the little pack would prove to be the most essential for this birth.

Leaving my husband and sleeping son in the home, I felt the spirit of adventure as I drove through the quiet streets. The light was just beginning to shift the darkness of the summer sky. My baby had been awake all night with me and was moving actively. I explained what was happening and caressed my belly, saying, "You are coming out into the world soon. These squeezes will help you move down through my body. Soon I'll hold you in my arms. I can't wait to see you."

Walking up to the labor and delivery desk on the hospital's third floor, carrying my small backpack, my mood shifted and I felt lonely. My husband would meet me here as soon as our son awoke and he could arrange care with the neighbors. Meanwhile, a nurse guided me to a spacious birthing room. I began to labor on my own.

My grandmother came to mind. Her stories of birth involved laboring alone, watching the clock until someone came in to medicate her. She was unconscious for both of her children's births—the births of my mother and uncle. I reminded myself that I would not be alone for this birth; my husband, midwife, and doula would be arriving soon. Setting my backpack onto a chair, I changed into a hospital gown. I decided to try the hot tub, where I entered transition with my first son, but it felt too hot. Instead, I paced around my birthing room.

The initial nurse, who was encouraging and warm, ended her shift. A new nurse came on. She began her shift by suggesting that we monitor my baby with an electronic fetal monitoring device. I sat on the bed and waited while she mechanically squirted cold gel onto my belly. I felt myself bristle at her touch. Not surprisingly, she had difficulty obtaining a reading. I peered into her face, observing her detachment from what she was doing. Then she barked an order at my baby. Directing her voice towards my belly she said, "Stop moving around!"

I caressed my belly protectively, guarding my space, startled by her demeanor that was so atypical of this hospital's thoughtful staff. I took the external monitor. "Let me do it," I responded sharply.

Placing the monitor on my own belly, I talked to my baby. "Let's just get a reading, honey." The strip of paper spat out from the electronic monitor. Barely looking at me, the nurse focused on the monitor strip. "This doesn't look like a pattern that resembles labor," she declared, and strode out of the room.

We'll see about that, I thought. Good thing I had brought my altar and energy tools. I spoke to my baby. "You just do whatever you need to; don't pay any attention to her. I'm going to clear the room and make it a sacred space."

Creating a Resonant Birth Field

I set to work, laying a cloth for the altar and covering it with special stones, herbs, and the birth necklace we created to welcome my baby. I put on Jennifer Berezan's CD *ReTurning*, a melodic chant recorded in an ancient cave, which I was drawn to during this baby's pregnancy. Then I sprinkled salt around the room, blessing our space as sacred and protected. In the blessing, I asked that all who enter rise to and resonate with the frequency of our vibration—noting inwardly that if this nurse did not change her tune, she would not be part of our birthing team.

After the room was blessed, the energy field was softer and more spacious. I walked across the room to turn up the birthing music and almost doubled over from the strength of a contraction. The nurse walked into the room at that moment. I felt myself regarding her, inviting forward a new pattern. She saw my response to the contraction and suggested that we check my cervix.

In hindsight, I am uncertain about all the monitoring and checking. Monitoring a woman during labor can often interfere with the flow of birth and tends to engage the cognitive or rational mind. Birth is an intuitive process that is more easily accessed by surrendering cognition.

The challenge with being monitored during birthing is that it is tempting to try to predict logically how far you have to go, but there is little logic in birth. The birth process can seem to stall, and the cervix will show less dilation progress, but perhaps the baby is resting or shifting position in a way that is not measurable. Alternately, birth can change pacing and move rapidly to complete dilation—particularly when a woman is following the intuitive flow in her body.

As the nurse now checked me, she found that my cervix had opened from three to six centimeters and the contractions were coming very strongly. Birth can progress contrary to the general rule of the suggested cervical dilation, which equates to one centimeter per hour. My cervical progression accelerated when my baby engaged more fully. This baby wanted a sacred space; he moved into the birth experience as soon as I reset the intentions in the room.

This shift in my birthing body, in response to aligning the energy field, conveyed how important it is to tend to the energy for birth—and yet it is so often missed. Birth is a sacred entry, and when the energy is aligned it can help to ease this process. The nurse responded to the energy setting in the room; she softened and held a more thoughtful presence. Later, I would hear from another nurse that she had been widowed the previous year and had been bearing a gruff demeanor ever since. I felt compassion for her. The birth and death doorways have much in common, one doorway in and another out. Perhaps coming into the birth field was stirring her grief.

Still, this was my baby's birth, and he deserved a sacred space. The birth field was ready; my baby could make his sacred entry.

Dropping into the Body

Within another half an hour, at about nine o'clock in the morning, my husband, my midwife Karen, and the doula arrived. The birth intensity ramped up. Still, though, I did not feel like my baby was moving down the birth canal. Having experienced birth before, I knew there was a natural progression of downward movement through the pelvis. Something did not quite feel right. My midwife confirmed that my baby was in a posterior position.

Weeks later, I would research posterior births online. A posterior birth means that the baby's face is toward the front of the pelvis, rather than face down in the more ideal anterior position. As mentioned previously, an anterior position is optimal because it facilitates the alignment necessary for the baby's head to move through the pelvic canal.

Recommendations for preventing a baby's posterior position and encouraging the anterior position include sitting upright rather than back on the pelvis during the last trimester of pregnancy. I had spent many hours of the previous two months slouched back on our couch, avoiding the summer heat and reading to my older son, and perhaps setting up a posterior birth position. During the birth, though, I only knew that the contractions were becoming much stronger and the birth was growing longer. My baby and I were tired. Still, the intensity increased.

I walked and rocked my hips. My baby's heart rate stayed strong. The hours passed. At about two o'clock in the afternoon, my midwife checked my cervix, and the opening was about eight centimeters. She suggested that we use Pitocin to increase the effectiveness of the contractions. Though I am a strong proponent of natural birth, I told her that I would need an epidural if we added any more stimuli to this birth. I felt as if I was beginning to slip beneath the wave after wave of contractions.

My beloved midwife suggested that everyone step out of the room and let me rest. Once alone, I instinctively put my head down and my bottom up, resting my head on my arms. I stopped trying and released all effort, surrendering to the moment. Deep and vast quiet surrounded me. And though I would not recognize it until later, this was the still point that I always met before my babies emerged. I felt something shift. Looking back, the position allowed my baby to turn a bit and engage farther into the canal. I started to groan, and Karen came back into the room. "She's at transition, and this baby's coming," I heard her say to the others.

As my son emerged, I felt a powerful sense of love from the whole birth team. We had worked so hard, my baby and I. Unlike the birth of my first son, where I had watched his entry with a mirror, I could not even open my eyes. It took every ounce of effort to ease him down through this ring of fire and into the world. I touched his head and, through my body, said a silent hello that only he would hear.

His brother was wet and slippery when he came through, like his watery Pisces sign, with dark eyes that reminded me of a seal. This baby's entry was hot and dry like the fire of a little Leo. Finally, with one last push, he arrived in the late afternoon. I took him onto my chest, and he made soft noises like a kitten.

"What a strong baby you are," I whispered to him. "I know you worked that whole time to come in. Thank you, sweet one. Now you can rest."

Practicing Loving Self-Acceptance

I had planned to let my newborn son crawl up my chest with support. Some birth experts suggest that we are wired for—and empowered by—this movement up the mother's belly to reach the breast and that it assists breastfeeding by orienting the baby to his mother's scent. But he was so worn out that I just placed him on the nipple. He took it right away and peeked out at the world with one bright blue eye half open. I saw a new lightness in the nurse who had been so gruff; she had stayed beyond her shift time.

Later, I phoned one of my girlfriends who had had three posterior births and an epidural each time. "Don't ever feel guilty again," I said in response to her frequently voiced regret. My experience with a posterior labor was significantly more difficult than when I labored with a baby in a more aligned position. With a natural and uninterrupted birth, there are a series of hormonal cascades that occur, providing an optimal setup for bonding and breastfeeding, as well as for receiving the energy of birth. However, the pain and fatigue of my second childbirth opened my eyes to the more intense physical challenges of a prolonged labor. Each birth is unique and accompanied by unexpected factors to contend with.

In my pelvic care practice, I have sat with many women who felt ashamed that their birthing experience required intervention or did not meet their expectations. We can prepare for our pregnancy, birthing, and mothering journeys, yet life may take us outside our plan. Creating a birth plan is a powerful exercise, as it allows you to set up a framework of intention and space for the new potential coming forth, but it does not control the experience. So create a framework but then surrender to the process and be compassionate with yourself at each step of the mothering journey.

There is an ocean of judgment around mothering and parenting, even from us as mothers. I remember watching harried moms at the preschool drop-off with my first child, wondering why they did not seem as present as I did at the time. Later I would recognize the frenzied preschool mother as one with multiple children to attend to. I would become one myself as I hurried between multiple drop-offs and pick-ups, multiple treat schedules and activities or assignments, and a multitude of expectations that became impossible to fully meet. Let's make an intention as women not to judge ourselves or one another. Judgment arises from a closed heart and a lack of understanding for the path of another. In birthing, mothering, and life, we do our best—and ideally we love ourselves and one another through the process.

The Energy of Labor and Birth

From an energy perspective, a woman approaches the opening of the spirit door near the end of pregnancy. This opening correlates with a point in time, approximately nine months after conception. But during the natural progression of labor, there is also a gradual expansion in her energy field that allows her to connect with and receive the birth energy through her body. In the case of birth interventions or cesarean, and particularly when labor is initiated by a surgery, this natural energy process is often incomplete, and a woman can benefit from the pelvic energy meditations for rebalancing the birth energy flow (as shown in chapter 5).

Since our organs and bodies imprint even early life experiences, the act of giving birth often stimulates dormant energies, particularly in the lower chakras (or energy centers) where the primary expansion takes place. Review the diagram of the wild feminine landscape: the physical and energetic space comprising the pelvic bowl (page 10). The physical structure of the pelvis lies in the center, layers of energy surround the bowl, and then the realm of spirit and the divine are part of the greater field.

When a woman conceives, spirit energy comes into her body from the greater realm. This sacred energy touches her womb space and settles with the fertilized egg in making her baby's body. While the pregnancy is gestating, there is a connection between spirit and body in the creation of life, which has led many cultures to celebrate pregnancy as a divine process.

Prior to labor, a woman's body begins to expand both physically and energetically. She may feel sensitive, as her boundaries are more fluid at this time. Reducing activity and avoiding crowds helps keep her energy field clear as her body opens to receive the energy for birth.

During labor, a woman's womb and pelvis expand, again both physically and energetically, to assist the passage of the baby down through her body and into the world. Her womb dilates, her pelvic muscles stretch, and her pelvic bones move apart. Likewise, her energy field expands to the point of making contact with the full spirit door and the greater energies of the spiritual realm. As this happens, the birth energy pours through her body and accompanies her baby into life. This flow of life is the thread between mother and child that serves as both an energetic bond and a place to access soul information. It also activates the external connection between a mother and child, which begins with in-arms care and breastfeeding. A mother's body awakens and responds to her child, offering the potential to relate to her body in a wholly expanded way.

Birth energy flow may be disrupted in a difficult or traumatic birth, causing mothers to feel that something is not right. In a cesarean birth, the natural energy process can be disrupted simply because of the intensity of surgery and its effects on the body and baby. Disruptions in the energy flow may also impact breastfeeding, because the energy current that assists the breastfeeding relationship is diminished. However, the birth energy flow that aligns mother and child can be reaccessed at any time, regardless of the difficulty of a birth event. It can even be transferred, as in the case of adoption. (Again, see the Restoring the Birth Energy Flow and Bond exercise in chapter 5 to learn more.)

Aligning Energy to Prepare for Birth

Connecting with the creative center of the pelvic bowl is a vital part of preparing for labor and aligning the core energy for birthing. By taking a birthing class, reading books, and learning about the labor process, a woman makes a framework of support for the labor and birth. Ultimately, however, it is the journey to the spirit door within herself, the physical and energetic opening within her center, that allows a mother to birth her baby. Her baby is also working in this same space to move and turn his or her body down and out into the world.

In honor of this deep energetic space of the body, where mother and child meet, I guide women through the following meditation approximately one month prior to their "due date." In this process of guiding pregnant women, though my hands only rest on their body and all our work is to contact the energetic space, the baby drums on the mother's belly as if to emphasize the wisdom and energy movement we encounter in the process.

Making a connection to the energetic space in the pelvic bowl prepares a woman to access the energy that opens the spirit door. Contacting this space before labor can assist the birth flow that will bring a woman's baby through this doorway and into the outer realm. It facilitates the process of clearing stagnant energies in the pelvic bowl, allowing her to receive more creative flow. This place can also be accessed in preparation for a cesarean birth or for guidance and support in any labor challenge. I went to this place in myself when my second son's labor was stalling, which inspired me to change my body position. Completely following an intuitive flow beyond my rational mind, I moved into a position that allowed my son to turn himself and continue his movement down the pelvic canal to be born. We can prepare for labor from this place, birth from this place, mother from this place, and create our lives from the bright essence of our own wise centers.

Exercise: Preparing the Spirit Door and Blessing the Birth Field

1. Bring your attention to your pelvic bowl. Say hello to your baby in the womb and communicate that you are preparing for his or her entry into the world. Mothers have a psychic or energetic ability to communicate with their children, particularly when a mother listens from her womb center. This begins when the baby is in the womb but continues after their birth as well and can be cultivated to assist the energy bond between mother and child. Babies also align with the mother; wherever your presence and focus is, they will join you there. To give birth vaginally and access the womb energy, it is helpful for you to connect with your creative core.

2. To work with the energy around the spirit door, close your eyes and, with your mind's eye, look to the front of your pelvic bowl. Sense into this space. What do you notice here? Are you ready to step into the birth process and mother this child? If there is any contraction or congestion in this area, feel the specific sensations. Ask if there is any message for your mothering or approaching birth. Breathe into this energy until it feels spacious and clear.

3. Repeat the same process to the right side of the pelvic bowl. This is the action-oriented masculine aspect of your energy field. Notice what is here for you. Are there any tasks for this focused energy to attend to? Receive the messages and align the energy on this right side so that your masculine aspect is ready to engage this adventure.

4. Continue toward the back of the pelvic bowl. What support is there for you in this birth process? Imagine the support you have cultivated and then rest back into this space, or make a note of the additional support that is needed in order for you to rest.

5. Now sense into the left side of your bowl. This is the dreamy and receptive feminine aspect of your energy field. Notice what is here for you. Sense into the expansive left side to receive the energy and inspirations you will need for this birth and time at the spirit door. Let yourself receive the blessings that will come.

6. Return to your center. Notice what has changed in the alignment and potential of your pelvic energy field. This is the space that will contain the spirit door. Your energy will expand into this space in order to birth your baby. Remember to access the greater energies of the spirit realm (like the outer ring of the wild feminine landscape) as support for both of you. When you call on spirit, you imagine the naturally aligning energies surrounding you, like a blossom-scented breeze or the warmth of sunlight.

7. In your sacred center, set an intention for the approaching birth. Send a wave of love to your baby. Then walk once

more around your pelvic energy field while blessing this space: *May we have a bountiful birth. May we be held and protected. May the energy be clear and aligned. May we receive the blessings of this journey together.* Whatever you wish to speak from your heart, let this love surround you as you travel to the spirit door to meet your baby.

Birth as Initiation

Prepare yourself for a journey just as you might for any great adventure. Gather your resources, not just for the pregnancy and birth but also for the time period of learning how to be a mother to your child. Imagine that you are traveling to a foreign country, because motherhood takes you into new land that life has scarcely prepared you for. Trying to read about having a baby is about as helpful as reading about another language in order to speak it. Instead, observe the mothers and children in your midst. Connect to your own body and listen to the ancient flow within for the guidance, information, and qualities you seek in mothering this new soul.

Make an extended time in the postpartum period for coming to know your baby and integrating the changes of mind, body, and spirit that accompany your journey into motherhood. Clear wide swaths of space from work and other obligations. There is so much focus on the pregnancy and birth experience. However, the nine to twelve months on the other side of the birth door require equivalent support for mother and baby to allow both to fully integrate the tremendous physical and energetic shifts that occur.

Pelvic Wisdom and Postpartum Care

After birthing, your pelvic tissues will be stretched and the vagina swollen. During birth, you can alleviate some of these stretch effects by taking a side-lying position rather than a full-upright one. Talk with your midwife or birth practitioner in advance about supporting your perineum with gentle counterpressure as the baby emerges.

Afterward, remain in bed as much as possible during the first two weeks to assist your recovery. Concentrated rest is vital for your long-term pelvic and energetic health. In your preparations, remember to anticipate the postpartum period and the need for rest after birthing. This stillness allows your body to heal and the birth energy to move through you. You can receive the birth energy current and all it contains for you and your child. Your baby can integrate the energy transfer into their body. After the wide opening in the field that occurs with birth, there is an extended period of weeks and even months where the spirit door closes and energy realigns.

●●

THE ENERGETICS OF THE SPIRIT DOOR

In the home birth of my third son, as the birth door opened, I was no longer contained in the borders of my body. My whole being was liberated by not having to limit myself to a hospital room or bed. Instead of the sterile hospital environment, I was comforted by the wood fire and the soft colors and morning light that surrounded me. Birth at home felt far more natural and satisfying on every level. My energy field shifted from where it rests just around my body to instead fill the whole room. At the moment of my son's birth, both his essence and mine were joined in the birth space as one, rather than moving as two separate spirits in two separate bodies. Our energies swirled and mixed, like light on water or clouds in the wind. I physically lifted him onto my chest and held him in my arms, but our energies moved all around us.

I carefully observed these birth patterns from the bedroom where my newborn and I spent the first two weeks. At one week after birth, our energies were still fluid, and expanded to fill about half the room. After two weeks, the energy was closer to our bodies. It was not until about three months that the energy felt more solidly shaped around my body, and my son and I had a more distinct energy boundary, though we still moved as one unit. The transfer of birth energy through the spirit door had occurred. We could be out in the world with less sensitivity.

Though many transitions occur after a birth event and it is easy to be distracted, focus attention on your body and your energy field. Notice the sensations you feel and your profound connection, in body and spirit, to your baby. Any challenges you encounter may invite growth or healing. By observing the subtle layers in this transition time, you will witness the miracle of spirit coming into body through the spirit door within your female form.

....

What blessings or energy have your received from your time at the spirit door?
How has birth energy transformed you or your family?
How would you like to access more of this potency?

Everyone Has a Place

Integrating a new baby into the family means finding a shared purpose and connection point, and also recognizing the place and value of every family member. With each new baby that joined our family, I made a nightly meditation, beginning with my connection to the baby and then including every person in our family. In my meditation, I tuned in to each person's unique essence, seeing each of us in my mind's eye and acknowledging the space that each one uniquely holds.

Depending on the ages or developmental stages of siblings, it can take some time for them to adjust to a new family member. Be aware that your journey to the spirit door and the intensity of the transition process may be unsettling for them. The intensity may also decrease your patience. Reassure them (and yourself) of your connection, with special bonding time and extra touches and hugs, and use their birth energy meditation to cultivate the mother-child energy bond as the family evolves. Reflecting this truth to our children, of the blessings they contain in relationship to others, helps them access and then bring their gifts to the world. The birth door brings a child's soul essence into being, but it is living with a family and community that teaches them how to engage this essence in relation to life.

What place does each member of your family hold?
How can both the family energy and individual expression be cultivated?

Love Is the Center, and So Are You

In our mothering tasks, our attention is often pulled outside ourselves, and yet we are the center for the family. Bringing focus back to the center and tending this place, we find a resonance with life from which our creative essence and the source of our mothering arises. Your creative energy is also for you to enjoy.

Tending to your own center as a mother while being called to take care of another can feel awkward. It takes time and patience to learn how to care for your creative self and balance that with the care of your family. To access your creative essence, you may find that you need a connection to the earth, a practice of ritual, ways to engage the deeper realms of spirit, or a daily experience of your unique expression. Try making a collage or bouquet or taking an art class. Being intentionally creative brings a vibrant energy into your center and home that illuminates new facets of your mothering.

Finding ways to channel a creative flow or a connection to spirit will refill your mothering well and expand the potential for your mothering. It also reminds you to honor your sacred beauty. When you live from the beauty of your own center, your children learn to live from theirs.

What do you need as a creative woman?
How will you incorporate this into your mothering life?

Unconditional Love for the Body: Embracing Your Changing Form

One practice of honoring yourself as sacred is to love your body even as you change form. Most women encounter body-image issues, even reexperiencing ones that may have been dormant, when their belly begins to bulge and their pregnant body becomes full and robust.

The first time I became pregnant, I was surprised to encounter my own body shame in response to my growing form. I went to my local goddess shop to purchase a divine feminine statue that was round and full-figured, and I began to say daily blessings for my body. This practice dispelled the negativity and helped me embrace the goddess within. I would need this practice again postpartum, when my body and vagina were swollen and my whole form altered, and again when I finished a decade of pregnancy and nursing to find that my breasts and body had transformed once more.

Honor yourself and all that your body has done in pregnancy, birth, and postpartum by countering any negative thoughts with blessings. For example, if you feel self-conscious about your weight, your stretched belly, or changes to your vagina, you might bless yourself: *I am sacred. May I know the blessing of my body. May my body be replenished. I give thanks for my body.*

Learning to love your body unconditionally is a good practice to prepare for the ongoing bodily changes that occur in parallel with your fertile center throughout your life, from the onset of menstruation until well after it ceases. Your body houses your spirit; it is a sacred place. By expanding your definition of self beyond your physical nature to include the beauty of your spirit, you ensure access to this potent creative mothering resource across time.

As a mother, you will feel vulnerable as you navigate body changes, partner shifts, and the demands of work and family each day. Sometimes you will bask in the blessings of your life, and sometimes you will struggle. Whenever you feel the most vulnerable, remember that you are worthy of love and a true blessing. Let the love flow to you—because love is the center, and so are you.

FOUR

After the Birth:
A New Way of Being

Two days after my first baby was born, I found myself at Babies "R" Us. Combine an excited first-time grandmother with a highly suggestible postpartum mom, and what ensued was a field trip to stock up on all things baby. I had never been to a baby-oriented megastore. The floor-to-ceiling display of bottles, carriers, cribs, strollers, toys, and other baby supplies was overwhelming to my sensitive postpartum nerves and energy system.

My pelvis throbbed, and I searched for a place to sit. Near a long line of cribs, I found a rocking chair, where I sat down and cried. Did I need all of this stuff? Of course not, but to a two-day postpartum new mom like me, I had no idea what was essential for embarking on this task of mothering and providing for my baby.

My hard-driving professional trajectory had prepared me well for forward motion, but I had no idea how to reconfigure my life for a baby's pace. Nor did I know that my own body would benefit from slowing down. The previous year, while working full-time, I had restored our hundred-year-old house with my husband, tackling enormous lists of errands and tasks around the edges of my work schedule. I thrived on action, so it was difficult to rest with the post-birth energy that coursed through my body, inspiring me to move. Days after giving birth, I was also surprised by the wall that I would suddenly hit out of nowhere. My energy would drop and tears would flood my eyes, or I would start to shake. I simply did not know that I needed to rest.

Two weeks later, my rancher mother-in-law came for a visit. She took one look at my shaking hands and tucked my baby and me into bed. Accustomed to the natural rhythms of living on a farm, she took naps on a daily basis. In fact, her family seemed to relish the downtime of naps interspersed with the work of each day. She spoke gently, "I'm just going to be real quiet and sit here in bed reading my newspaper. Let's close the blinds and you can lie down."

Surrendering to her wise counsel, I climbed into bed and laid my head on the pillow next to my sleeping baby. I breathed in his scent, my eyes resting on his beauty just before they closed into sleep. So began my first relationship with rest, first somewhat guiltily and then eventually as a window of retreat to be savored. I had been hungry for this permission to stop doing and just be. After her visit, my family and I began our own daily ritual of afternoon naps and quiet time that would serve us well for more than a decade of parenting.

The Other Side of the Spirit Door

After giving birth, you will feel yourself a changed woman. In the days following the birth of a baby, a profound transformation occurs in your body, being, and psyche. This change can feel exhilarating and overwhelming at the same time. You have passed through the spirit door with your child. You have also stepped into motherhood, a formative process with every child you have.

After birth, there is a tremendous physical shift as your womb continues to shed blood and fluids for many weeks. Your body may feel stretched and worn by the pregnancy and birth while also feeling simultaneously energized. Vaginally, you can feel newly aware of this space or a bit disconnected. Many mothers feel worried about the changes in their body, while others may be too distracted by the life changes to notice themselves. Either way, when you try to do a Kegel (squeezing your pelvic floor muscles) after giving birth, these muscles can seem quite weak, as if you can hardly engage them. This weakness occurs because the muscles are stretched in the process of giving birth. With this stretch effect, the muscles' set points of engagement are literally farther apart (think of a stretched rubber band that has less elasticity).

Pelvic muscles can also be bruised and sore from the impact of birth. The muscles will begin to repair themselves, but since you also need your body's reserves for rebalancing the womb and pelvis post-birth as well as making milk, muscle recovery can be a slow process. After my first birth experience, I experienced vaginal pain from a few post-birth stitches and required direct massage from a women's health physical therapist in order to heal. This personal experience motivated my later women's health practice focus on supporting women's pelvic care during the postpartum period.

After my first birth, I also remember my confusion as I went to put on my favorite pair of overalls. I was surprised to find them tight and uncomfortable. I thought that once I had given birth I would be instantly smaller, perhaps like my former self. My vagina felt swollen and tender; my belly was stretched from the pregnancy and my still-enlarged uterus.

Our female bodies are amazing, and they deserve our patience while recovering from all that they do for us in pregnancy, birth, and mothering. The womb requires about six to eight weeks to return to a pre-pregnancy form, and the swollen tissues of the vagina need to heal. Meanwhile, the hormones and body fluids readjust from the pregnant state of nourishing two bodies to that of the postpartum and nursing body. This is a major transformation that ought to be acknowledged.

Most women find that, after the initial postpartum changes, their body continues to evolve and change over the entire post-birth year. Major shifts occur at three, six, nine, and twelve months postpartum, concurrent with the baby's developmental changes. Also, with prolonged nursing, a woman will find additional changes in her body that correspond to each change in the nursing pattern, which gradually tapers over time. Upon moving through the intensity of the postpartum year, a woman may finally return her awareness to healing herself. (There is detailed information for addressing postpartum effects in chapter 6.)

The energy that emerges most powerfully at birth also continues to move through your body for at least three months postpartum. As during menstruation, when your energy field is more open to clear your center, the post-birth energy field opens even more widely to allow in the energy of another soul. Look at your beautiful baby and notice how he or she has an ethereal, almost otherworldly radiance, especially during the first three months while your baby's essence gradually comes into his or her body. This visible spirit energy around babies is the magic they bring to remind us of the everyday sacred.

There is a movement from spirit into body, and each one of us embodies it in this way. Even if you are adopting a child, you can hold an energetic space for this energy transfer for your child (see the exercise Restoring the Birth Energy Flow and Bond, page 118).

This energetic transfer requires an expansion in your center that may cause you to feel vulnerable and easily off-balance, which is why mothers and babies are commonly encouraged to stay close to the home and bed during this time. Cherish your downtime and witness the amazing potential of this energy dance between your baby and your female body.

....

PHYSICAL AND ENERGETIC SHIFTS

Here are some of the physical and energetic shifts you may experience or witness after the birth of your baby.

0 to 3 Months
- Baby is coming into his or her body, literally embodying the life energy that came in with birth.
- Mother is healing and restoring her body from birth, making milk, and becoming a mother.
- Her mothering lineage comes alive. Partnership and whole family shifts.
- Energy is transferring through the spirit door in the mother's body to baby. (If baby is adopted, this transfer can be cultivated energetically at any point.)

3 to 6 Months
- Baby is becoming more aware of the world and his or her own body.
- Energetic transfer from birth door is more complete.
- Mother and baby are finding their rhythm together.
- Mother is primary source of nourishment and comfort.
- Mother and baby still move as one energy body.

6 to 9 Months
• Baby is beginning to explore movement and actively engage with others and the world.
• Nourishment is shifting from primarily milk to food.
• Mother may begin to feel the beginning of return to her own body but is still primary anchor for her baby (energetically and physically).

9 to 12 Months
• Baby begins initial awareness of being separate from mom.
• Mother's body begins to restore itself from the nine months on the other side of the birth.
• Mother and baby continue the life learning they will share in this journey.
• Energy connection continues to flow between mother and baby, and they draw upon this potential to learn, grow, and explore their expanding world.

....

Integrating the Changes
Learning to heal and address your needs in the midst of taking care of a baby is an entirely new skill set. You are discovering this new person who now lives in your home. As witnessed by parents of multiple children, each baby is a unique individual with unique ways of being. Reading your baby's cues and finding a rhythm together is an organic process that happens day by day. Until you are experienced, it is difficult to explain the transformation that occurs as you reorient around this new soul who is coming into his or her own body and the beginning of life.

It is normal to feel a range of emotions as a mother, from buoyant euphoria to tears of sadness or distress. Grief is an emotion that accompanies all transitions, even those we are anticipating, because it assists us in shedding that which no longer serves us in order to remake ourselves for the way forward.

In addition to the pelvic rebalancing required after birthing, some of the pregnancy and nursing hormones continue to make your ligaments—the bands that support the connections between the bones and joints—more lax. Stretched pelvic and abdominal muscles, combined with lax ligaments, mean that you are more vulnerable to strain or injury. The uterine ligaments that support the position of your uterus are also vulnerable to strain, particularly in the first three to six months postpartum.

The potential for injuring or depleting your already overtaxed postpartum body is another reason to stay close to bed for at least six to eight weeks. Avoid lifting anything heavier than your baby; even though you can lift something, it does not mean you should. Your postpartum and nursing body is vulnerable and must restore itself from the nine-month process of holding and growing the body of another. Lie down several times per day. Avoid all strenuous exercise; take short walks. Preserve your long-term pelvic health and core vibrancy by lying down and staying down. Store your energy as if preparing for the winter, the postpartum year is a marathon of healing, milk-making, and core transformation.

Now that you are on the other side of the spirit door, it is time to integrate all the physical, energetic, and spiritual changes that have occurred for you as well as to build a new relationship with your baby and partner.

Making a Postpartum Care Plan

For reasons that will now be clear, my primary advice for new mothers is to REST: Reduce Energy and Slow Time. In our busy modern world, there is a clear lack of rest, and most women have not developed the skill of resting. Birth also brings an energy flow and excitement that can make it difficult to rest, yet that energy is meant to sustain the early period of baby care.

Rest means lying down several times during the day and sleeping when your baby sleeps, especially in the first three months. Rest means slowing down enough to find that state of inner stillness where cells are replenished. Slow time means doing less. Let the housework go or hire help, reduce your standards for what can be done, let your partner run errands to the store, and clear anything that is nonessential. Make the postpartum period into a home-based retreat; read, journal, take baths, taste food, and savor the dream time.

Having a baby opens your creativity, and resting allows you to ponder and dream in the midst of the creative flow. Vast quiet allows you to hear your baby and connect with his or her soul essence. Many women receive visions or insights regarding the family or their creative future during this fluid time. The postpartum mind is less detail oriented and more intuitive; in fact, details can often escape your awareness, but your general creative capacity is robust. Meditating and journaling are powerful tools for capturing the essence of the postpartum creative flow. Just keep in mind that taking action on these dreams is at least one to two years away, when you are through the initial intensity of caring for your baby.

Presently, how are you resting and slowing down? How would you like to add more rest?

What dreams or visions are coming to you? What are you sensing from your baby?

Are there any areas that need more support or care?

Caring for Your Body after Birthing a Baby

Take care of your body after the intensity of birthing a baby. Gather your support, receive massage or bodywork, engage the body with light exercise while avoiding vigorous exercise, and use good body mechanics that include aligned postures and positions throughout the day.

Many women begin to exercise in the postpartum period. I caution against exercising because, again, your body is vulnerable both postpartum and while nursing. With the combination of fatigue from less sleep, the demands from nursing, and the lax ligaments from hormones, your body is already challenged and not well-positioned for vigorous exercise. In fact, you can cause permanent strain to your pelvic organs by engaging in high-impact exercise during this vulnerable time. Once you are sleeping more and nursing less, and at least nine months past the birth, exercise can be incorporated, but still ought to be done with awareness of the postpartum body's needs.

Taking brief walks is an ideal postpartum exercise, and you can build up distance as your body feels stronger. If you have any pelvic heaviness, pressure, or other pelvic symptoms, it is ideal to reduce any stress and see a pelvic care practitioner to restore pelvic alignment as soon as possible. This pelvic pressure is a sign that your pelvic muscles are not able to support you through your day, and they can be strained further if not addressed. Pelvic heaviness may also occur when you are overly fatigued, signaling the need for rest. (Chapter 6 discusses pelvic support for healing your postpartum body.)

It is normal to feel nervous about having sex the first time after having a baby. Proceed slowly, but do try to make love with your partner. Sex is nourishing and healing, assuming it is not overly painful. (Chapter 6 discusses pelvic healing and receiving pelvic care to ensure your return to full sexual pleasure.) Sex is a wonderful pelvic massage that clears stagnation and increases flow. Though the postpartum focus is mostly on the baby, children benefit immensely from the flow of energy in a robust parental relationship. Tending to the love that strengthens your partner connection ensures a strong family as well.

....

RECIPE FOR POSTPARTUM CARE

1. Rest
- Go to bed early, and take a daily nap.
- Alternate light movement with rest throughout the day.
- Conserve energy for recovering and bonding with your baby.
- Alternate action with rest to pace yourself and refuel yourself each day. Just taking care of your baby and nursing is a tremendous expenditure that requires daily replenishment.

2. Support healing
- Wear a pelvic wrap. Wrap a cloth around your pelvis or wear a belly band to provide extra support while you are up during the day. This helps the pelvis feel more contained even while the ligaments have laxity.
- Do daily sitz baths as needed. Soaking the perineum in warm salt water will improve circulation.
- Contact a medical provider immediately with any excessive bleeding or fever.
- Eat well-balanced meals, with frequent fluids and snacks to nourish yourself. Love and honor your body.
- Cherish this sacred time; receive the birth energy.
- Leave the housekeeping and shopping to others when possible; gather your support.
- If you had a cesarean, wear the AbdoMend C-section Recovery Kit wrap.

3. Receive bodywork
- At two months postpartum, receive vaginal massage from a pelvic care practitioner. Skilled massage is beneficial for

restoring fascial and organ alignment, improving muscle balance and engagement, and supporting overall cellular flow. Though I generally recommend vaginal self-massage, I would not suggest attempting to heal postpartum effects with your own massage.

• Receive general bodywork, massage, and/or acupuncture to assist overall body balance and health. Engage in gentle sex when you are ready to enhance the flow of blood and chi.

• Postpartum depression can have a mechanical component partially caused by physical imbalance in the cranial-sacral fascia. Find a skilled cranial-sacral practitioner and acupuncturist to assist the body in returning to balance. It can also be the result of unhealed trauma that has been restimulated by the birth event or an inability to integrate the vast changes that have occurred. Both call for a multidisciplinary approach.

• Pubic symphysis separation is a strain or actual separation of the pubic connection in the pelvic ring. It requires rest, a pelvic belt, and a skilled bodywork practitioner.

4. **Reengage pelvic and abdominal muscles**

• Do ten to fifteen Kegel contractions of the pelvic muscles twice per day to improve blood flow and muscle mobility and to reset the pelvic floor.

• While standing, pull in lower abdominals (as a light belly squeeze) five to ten times to remind the lower belly muscles how to reset after the stretch of pregnancy. (Avoid sit-ups or crunches, which can strain abdominals.)

• Only lift something as heavy as your baby. (With older children, try to sit down and have them come to you rather than lifting them.) Engage pelvic and abdominal muscles when lifting your baby or to stabilize yourself while getting into or out of bed or a car.

- Use the Tupler Technique, a combination of an abdominal brace and a set of effective exercises designed to repair the diastasis recti (a split in the abdominal muscles) but is also helpful for the general abdominal stretch and loose belly effects of pregnancy. Take care of your body.

5. **Incorporate good body mechanics**
   - Use caution with lifting or doing too much the first year postpartum and as long as you are nursing. To increase core stability, engage the pelvic floor and abdominals during transition movements.
   - Practice good body mechanics by lifting and moving with intention and alignment. (Use the stroller when fatigued.)
   - Avoid sitting your baby on your hip and pushing your hip out to create a shelf, as this strains the pelvis. Instead, shift your weight onto one side and hold your baby with your arms. If your arms fatigue, switch sides. If they fatigue again, it is time to sit down and rest.

6. **Add gentle exercise routines**
   - To preserve long-term pelvic health, refrain from running, jumping, and intensive exercise regimes until you are one year postpartum.
   - Walking, yoga, and swimming are all good for restoring body balance without straining your postpartum body. Always listen to your body and modify your routine as needed.
   - When you have a sleepless night with your baby, do less and rest more to restore your body's reserves. An increase in pelvic prolapse or other pelvic symptoms often indicates core fatigue.
   - Gently stretch your body. Yoga has many helpful poses for stretching tired and tight muscles that result from carrying your baby and holding prolonged nursing positions.

....

Cherishing Yourself

In addition to taking care of your body, cherishing yourself is paramount. You are the center for your baby, and the way you feel impacts your child's well-being. Mothering is physically and emotionally demanding. Adding a new family member is a tremendous transition for everyone in the home. Attending to your physical, energetic, emotional, and general wellness is the key to sustained mothering. The more you attend to your needs and the well-being of your own center, the more balanced you and the family will be.

Women may either exercise due to fear about the changes in their body or, alternatively, ignore the body altogether. Again, rest, nutrition, and short walks are the best tools for helping the body to heal and realign postpartum. By attuning to the body rather than reacting to it, we ensure a caring approach rather than a fearful one. When we care for our body and cherish this center point of our mothering, we establish a positive body relationship that allows us to draw on our core resources. Our babies are profoundly connected to our body; our positive relationship with ourselves will greatly enhance these positive associations for our children.

Listening to Your Own Center

Before having our children, my best friend and I thought that becoming mothers might go well with obtaining doctoral degrees because we imagined our long, carefree days with a sleeping infant. We now laugh at our misconception, having been through the intensity of an infant's round-the-clock feedings, a time when taking a shower and feeding ourselves seemed like a victory for the day. In the emphasis on career development, there is an absence of knowledge about what it takes to care for children or our own inner lives. Though it is ideal to have an extended postpartum period that focuses on baby care and honing mothering skills, most people are not aware of the planning required to leave the professional realm for a prolonged period.

I intended to return to work for twenty-four hours per week when my first son was three months old. Three months was the longest time I'd ever been away from work in my adult working life, so this seemed like a luxury. And twenty-four hours seemed a brief workweek compared to my full-time schedule. But I had no idea how deep and visceral the mother-baby bond is, or that at three months, I would only have left him for a two-hour stretch of time—quite a bit less than my typical nine-hour workday. After some soul searching, I chose not to return to work as I had known it. My child had called me back to my center, and from the center I eventually wove a life and work-family balance that would support us.

There are many decisions to weigh at every stage of parenting, and every mother-child pair is different. Whether you are navigating work structures, daily routines, bed-sharing, baby-wearing, nursing patterns, bottle use, deciding how long to nurse, how to parent, and so on, it is important to make decisions from the wisdom of your center. Though co-sleeping has come into fashion, some families do better with cribs at night. The most essential piece is that everyone has a good sleep. I wore all my children in carriers and baby slings but also recognized that in other cultures baby-wearing is shared by the extended family and that I needed to use a stroller or set my baby down at times to rest myself. There is no definitive right or wrong way to do things, and every mother-child pair and family has to figure out what works for them.

Read about parenting techniques and talk to other parents to learn more regarding the various work-life options. In the end, however, sense what feels right in your body and family flow. Attune to your center and mother from there.

How has your life been remade by mothering?
How are you being called back to the center?
How will you build a more sustainable mothering
  life?

Taking Care of You: A Loving Daily Practice

To have the energy for mothering, it is vital to attend to yourself as a daily practice. One of my favorite daily self-care rituals is my cup of tea. I have a cup of tea in the afternoon and promise to drink it before it becomes cold. In order to do this, I have to stop doing or caretaking and focus on drinking the tea.

If my children ask me for something during this teatime, I tell them I am taking a moment for myself. They know that I take a cup of tea every day as a way to tend to myself, so they expect this. They may sit quietly with me or play nearby, but they also know that I will not do anything else until my tea is finished.

Even if I have work to do, I pause for my tea break, resisting the urge to multitask during this time. Instead I sit by the window and talk to my birds or notice the colors of the sky. This is a pause to refill the well for all that I do in the name of mothering and creating. I take in the moment and savor whatever it brings. I invite you to do the same. A small effort made daily adds up over the years. May all mothers and creative women take time to nurture themselves each day.

Your self-care as a mother has to come first so that you may replenish all that you give while mothering. Take care of yourself from the beginning. Recognize the energy you are expending even in gestating and birthing a child. Nursing further draws on your inner reserves and caretaking continues for decades—longer if you have more than one child. Be aware of your place in the center. Care for yourself and store up your energy; when in need of these reserves, you will be glad you did.

Breasts and Breastfeeding: Refueling Your Fire

One of the first skills to learn with your baby is breastfeeding. Breastfeeding is not only nourishment but also an intimate way of communicating with your baby. Just hearing the cry of their newborn, many women will find that the milk in their breasts "lets down" or begins to flow. Breastfeeding also provides essential immunity to your baby and is the best preventative measure for any illness your child may have while building his or her immunity.

Early on, establish multiple breastfeeding positions to prevent strain on your body and to more efficiently empty milk from the breasts. Learn to breastfeed lying down in order to rest more fully while nursing. As you breastfeed your newborn, take the time to place rolled blankets or pillows around you and make a relaxed position for yourself so that you can rest your arms and shoulders. Maintain good alignment with nursing positions to provide support for your body and prevent fatigue. Keep your baby close and use skin-to-skin contact to facilitate the energy connection and subtle communication between your bodies. Also, position your baby for a good nipple latch to prevent nipple soreness. A nurse or midwife can observe your nursing pattern to provide specific instruction. Each baby will nurse differently. Finding direct, hands-on nursing support is essential in the first few hours and again in the next few days when it comes to ensuring that your baby has a good latch and is obtaining sufficient milk. Breastfeeding is an art and a skill that is best learned with an experienced lactation specialist right from the start.

As your baby grows, the breastfeeding becomes quicker and the baby can move his or her body toward the breast, so positioning is not as essential. However, using good body mechanics (positions that create the least strain) while lifting or caregiving goes a long way in maintaining your postpartum health. (Remember not to lift anything heavier than your baby.)

Breastfeeding can be challenging for multiple reasons. There can be judgment from others about breastfeeding, especially with nursing older children, because breasts may be seen as sexual. Unfortunately, there is confusion between sexuality and sensuality. Sexuality is the lovemaking that happens between consenting adults. Sensuality can play a role in sexuality but encompasses a much broader range of connection through the senses: walking barefoot on the grass is sensual, chocolate melting in your mouth is sensual, skin-to-skin contact with your baby is sensual. Being clear about the difference between sexuality and sensuality is helpful when others may impose their lack of clarity on the intimate space between mothers and children. Observe a child breastfeeding and notice their pleased expression; being held and nourished in this way is a sensual experience. Allowing our children to have nurturing sensual experiences will positively affect their bodily connection and provide the healthy foundation for their adult relationships and sexuality.

If you are having ongoing problems with breastfeeding, your baby may benefit from cranial-sacral treatments. This is a type of osteopathic bodywork that can enhance the fascial alignment in the cranial-sacral system, helping a baby feel more at peace in their body as well as to have a better latch and suck reflex. I know many mothers whose baby's nursing improved markedly with cranial-sacral treatments by a practitioner trained to work with infants. Maintaining milk production also requires replenishing yourself with fluids and healthy foods throughout the day.

If your baby is crying incessantly, he or she may not be receiving adequate milk due to overall supply or latch issues. Babies should be gaining weight steadily and filling out with milk fat. For one of my clients, a handheld scale misread the weight of her baby, so the baby's weight loss was missed. If a baby is lean and crying, it is likely the milk is not being taken in, and the solution requires assessment and potentially supplementation. It can be emotionally challenging to supplement with formula. Milk banks (supplied by the donated milk of other mothers) are an option. One way or another, it is vital for the baby to receive those early nutrients and essential fats.

Another interesting connection I have observed in my women's health practice is that between ovarian energy and breast milk. When I engage women in a pelvic meditation to increase ovarian energy, nursing moms will often feel their breast milk let down. Likewise, women with less energetic connection to one of the ovaries typically have less milk in the breast on that same side of the body.

One of my clients shared that increasing her connection and energy presence to her left ovary increased milk production in her left breast. When she pumped, she noticed that her left breast routinely made half as much milk as the right. Once she began working with her left ovary and feminine presence in the left energetic field, her breasts produced the same amount of milk.

Ovarian and breast health also relate to how you access your creative flow and nurture yourself. If you overuse your energy or give more than you receive, the breasts and ovaries will be less healthy energetically and physically. A breast infection is a sign of depletion and indicates the need to refill your energy wells. *Wild Feminine* contains many ovarian exercises as well as more detailed information regarding the right ovary and its relation to the masculine energy field and the left ovary and its connection to the feminine energy field. Below is one of my favorite breast/ovarian exercises to fuel your inner fire.

Exercise: Breast and Ovary Meditation to Fuel Your Fire

1. Bring your attention to your pelvic bowl and the source of your inner fire. You are a radiant and fertile being; sense this bright potential within.

2. First send a breath toward your left ovary. Blow on this ovary as you would a hot coal. As you breathe, ignite the fire in your left energy field. Sense the expanding warmth in this space. This is the feminine ovary, your inner muse and source of inspiration or nourishment. Have you been tending her? Ask how she might like to be inspired. Make a place for her energy and for tending her fire in your daily life.

3. Now send a breath toward your right ovary. Again, blow on this ovary as you would a hot coal. As you breathe, ignite the fire in your right energy field. Sense the expanding warmth in this space. This is the masculine ovary, your visible expression and spirit of adventure. Have you been accessing her energy in ways that fuel her fire? Ask what directions call to her presently. Carry her radiance into each day.

4. Return to your center and notice how your inner fires have changed. Are they brighter? Warmer? More vibrant? Breathe the warmth from these fires into your full energy field and to both breasts. Sense this breath, warmth, and love within. Nourish yourself with your fire before feeding others.

5. Tending your inner fire is essential for making an inspired life. Whether mothering or embarking on other creative ventures, the fire within is the fuel that will light your way. Give thanks for these fires and regularly tend their flames.

Sustaining a Long-Term Breastfeeding Relationship

Maintaining a long-term breastfeeding relationship required that I respect my body's need for nightly rest. After about a year of "on demand" or "whenever they wanted" nursing, I stopped all-night nursing. In this way, my babies and I were able to co-sleep but also have a fully rested night. I explained to each child that we would not be nursing during the night so that we could both get more sleep. When they awakened to nurse, I held them while they cried, continuing my firm but gentle mantra that we needed to sleep now and nurse in the morning. While providing comfort, I connected with them from the assured peace in my center.

Each of my children was different in learning the new nursing pattern. One son cried long and hard for almost an hour but then slept the rest of the night. My other two sons woke several times during the night, crying for just minutes on each occasion. But all three learned relatively quickly to accept the new pattern. When my children were ill, I made an exception to my "no night nursing" policy. While sick with any illness, they could again nurse on demand as needed. When they were well, I waited a night to transition and then said, "Now that you are feeling better, we need to stop nursing at night so we can have our sleep." Each child readjusted quickly.

I have had clients who kept nursing through their own exhaustion, and often their resentment grew until they stopped nursing altogether. Mothering in a balanced manner means listening to and working from our own center, which will give signs when we are becoming depleted and off-balance. Remember that nursing is part of a relationship, and the nursing pattern must feel good to you.

Finding a Sustainable Mothering Pace

Even though my mother-in-law taught me the importance of rest in the weeks after my first baby was born, I would not really slow down and fully attune to my center until one month after my son's birth, when I learned a difficult lesson. I was on a long walk with my son when I tripped and fell on the sidewalk. Looking back at one month postpartum, I should have still been staying near the bed. But instead, I took a forty-block walk with my son in a front carrier. After an hour of walking, I tripped and fell, hitting my son's head on the concrete.

My son had a skull fracture. (Note: He is now a strapping and fearless twelve-year-old.) We went by ambulance to the hospital, and a trauma team of fourteen specialists gathered around his tiny body and eventually concluded that his hairline fracture was stable. Now we had to rest, by doctor's orders, and the shock of the experience shifted me out of my tendency to push everything—an unbalanced, masculine pattern—toward a more feminine state of being. In *Wild Feminine*, I share my journey toward understanding the feminine essence. I eventually found that accessing the feminine requires that we be sufficiently present in the center in order to allow this beauty to unfold in our lives. Continuously moving or doing makes it difficult to connect with this center point where the feminine essence resides.

Though my exploration regarding the feminine spanned the next decade of my mothering life, my journey began the night after falling with my baby. It was a spiritual awakening, lying in the dark and listening to his breathing through the night. The first night was the most crucial, as we awaited the effects of the fall on his body.

Being in a more conventional hospital than the one where he was born, the medical team on the pediatric trauma ward insisted he be placed in the crib for an overnight observation period rather than in a bed with me. Pulling a chair next to him, I draped my body over the crib rail and embraced his tiny form. At last they put a cot for me next to the crib, and I lowered the side rail on the crib as far as it would go so that the cot and crib felt more like a bed. After we established this "bed" for my baby and me, my husband went home to attend to our young German shepherd, Kiva. I curled my body around my sleeping baby, instinctively knowing the healing power of the connection between us.

I felt comforted by a presence; spirit was there with me. I prayed through the night, and so many thoughts passed through my mind. A deep shift began to take place in my center. Though the fall was a deep shock, I felt that it was a tremendous gift. It illuminated the unconscious way I was still running my energy system in overdrive.

In the dark hours of the night, a nurse lifted my son into my arms. He slept soundly and nursed well. In the dawn light, his eyes opened to find mine. He smiled at me, his first face-to-face smile. His dark eyes were so bright. I breathed a deep sigh of relief and rested back against the cot. My cheeks wet with tears, I kissed his soft lips and whispered, "Thank you, thank you," speaking to him, to spirit, to the potential of each moment, to the angel that comes when you least expect it.

A Healing Journey

The effects of the fall on my son motivated me to seek out a gifted healer, a chiropractor and psychotherapist who worked with trauma in babies. She helped me heal the effects of the fall, like the tightness in his chest from the impact and the restrictions in his cranial system, which the Western medical system suggested might require surgery at some point. I then studied with her for two years.

In the process of learning the infant bodywork process she had developed, I began to heal some of the early patterns in my own body and energy field that kept me in a "doing" mode rather than a "being" mode, like keeping busy to avoid my feelings or staying productive in order to maintain a sense of value. Tapping into these stored feelings allowed me to clear my emotional container. Realizing I could channel joy in my center instead of using it as a storehouse for unresolved feelings, I altered the very place I mothered from. In this process of discovery, I also found an inner value and abundant creative flow that gave birth to a body of work and continues to nourish my family and me.

Having a child invites you to slow down and be in the moment. Postpartum energy is not meant to propel you into the world but rather to sustain you through rebuilding your body and creating a milk supply. It supports the early period of little sleep and much work. Growing a baby in the first year requires a tremendous outpouring of energy. The first year also calls for a whole new skill set and requires the transition from the pace of a production-oriented culture and a life built on achievement or professional development to one that is less visible, non-quantifiable, and focused on the home.

It is not just the children but also the feminine who calls us to the home and to a relationship with our core selves and our state of being. The feminine relies on our ability to retreat and find a still point; it is an inspired place of retreat from which all creativity arises. However, you may need to address past wounds before this inner space feels nourishing. Follow your children's lead to create a new path that is both productive and soul-filled. Falling with my son was a hard way to learn, but I can attest to the richness of a life that is built around the home, the center of life and family, and a more sustainable pace of living.

FIVE

The Healing Power of Birth Energy

Birth is a profound event, for the one being born and the one birthing, as well as those gathered to assist the process. Birth events are particularly impactful for the mother and baby simply because the experience imprints deeply in their bodies and in the energy of the mother-child bond. With the expansion in a mother's body and the openness of the newborn's energetic field, the birth event creates a sensitivity that can imprint either its potency or its challenge, depending on how it occurs. Even a relatively smooth birth may feel traumatic if it happens too rapidly, because there is not enough time for mom or baby to process what is happening.

If a birth is traumatic to the mother, she may talk about the birth in an attempt to rectify what feels imbalanced to her. Those around her may, with good intentions, suggest that she focus on the fact that she has a healthy baby and encourage her to set aside her feelings of unease. Yet if the birth energy flow has been disrupted in the trauma, a mother will not feel settled until the energy has been restored. She is fixated on the birth story in her desire for resolution; however, though the story alone will not heal the birth, it can provide clues to where the birth energy became disrupted.

The birth itself contains powerful energy medicine to address any imprints of trauma. This healing power of birth energy is potent because birth imprints set the stage for a baby's sense of the world, the family bond, and a woman's capacity for mothering or accessing her creative essence. Addressing an initial disruption at the spirit door, by restoring alignment in the body and birth field, ripples out with positive effects that layer into many aspects of life. We can access the birth field after a difficult labor to bring the necessary healing.

Healing Traumatic and Unexpected Birth Experiences

When birth is natural and uninterrupted, there is a tangible flow of energy through the mother's body that carries her child into life. This river of birth energy can be sustained to nourish mother and child through all the stages of their bond. A mother who has a difficult or even traumatic birth may feel like something is not right for her. Her child was delivered, but the energy flow likely was disrupted in the birth process.

In my work with women, my most potent revelation from the female body is that the birth energy flow can be recovered even after a disruption has occurred. No matter the age of the child or the time that has passed since a birth event, that river of birth energy can be restored. The birth energy is often still held within the mother's body. Working with a woman's energy field, she can reaccess the birth energy flow, reestablishing this connection point between her and her child.

The birth energy flow can be disrupted by medical intervention such as a cesarean, an epidural, vacuum extraction, or the removal of a retained placenta. It can be affected by postpartum hemorrhage or if the baby needs resuscitation. Likewise, if the mother is transported during the birth process, has a difficult relationship with the labor team, or becomes particularly exhausted in a prolonged labor, the energy flow can be disrupted. While intervention or transport may be necessary and even lifesaving, the process of intervention still alters the natural flow. However, though the physical aspect of the birth is complete, again, these disruptions can still be repaired by reaccessing the birth energy.

Not all birth intervention disrupts the energy flow, and assessing this disruption depends less on the story of the birth and more on the mother's postpartum perspective. If she feels generally at peace, the birth energy is likely flowing. If anything is troubling her about the birth or some aspect of the birth, or if she is having difficulty transitioning in the postpartum period or connecting with her child, then likely the birth energy field and flow are affected and in need of realignment. Simply talking about her experience will not bring resolution; rather she needs an energy medicine approach to restore the birth energy flow.

The Energy in Undisturbed Birth: The Birth Field

To understand the energy flow in an undisturbed birth, picture the wild feminine landscape (page 10) with a series of concentric rings that show the physical body surrounded by the energy field and then by the energy of spirit. As an energy reader, I see how birthing expands the pelvis and womb, both physically and energetically, into the realm of spirit in order to receive the life essence of a new being. In the natural process, birth and the opening of the spirit door create a radiant energy pattern like a multidimensional crystal. This pattern is the birth energy field.

When the birth energy field is established, the energy flows with the baby through the mother's womb and into life. This energy continues to flow as the baby lies on the mother's chest, taking the first breaths and then drinking her breast milk. This powerful current composes the energetic bond between mother and child for all of life. The birth energy is there to help them understand one another. If a mother knows how to access this energy, she will gain information and resources specific to mothering this child. Though a father or partner will form a deep parenting bond as well, much of the support for these family bonds arises in this birthing energy.

The Energy in a Disrupted Birth Process

When the birth process is disrupted, the birth field may never find its full expression. In this case, the birth energy is often interrupted or held within the womb, on the other side of the spirit door. This holding pattern in the body makes it challenging for a woman to integrate the birth event or access the energy of the birth. However, this birth imprint can be changed at any point in time, even long after the birth. Though we desire a beautiful birth experience, because of circumstances outside a woman's control, a birth event may not resemble her desired experience. It is a myth that if a woman simply does everything right, the birth will go according to her plan. Likewise, if a birth is difficult or traumatic, a woman may unnecessarily blame herself or wonder what she did wrong. I value the emphasis on natural birth that motivates women to make a birth plan and set the stage for a beautiful experience, yet I want all mothers to feel included in the blessing potential of birth energy, regardless of how the birth unfolds, and to release themselves from the burden of needing to achieve a particular birth event.

With intention and focus, a birth with intervention can also be a sacred process. For example, a woman can stay present in her body even as she receives an epidural. She can bring the sacred with her in a home-to-hospital transport and align the energy around her with simple blessings. Likewise, she can communicate to the baby in her belly about the intention for a planned cesarean.

In a natural birth, the baby is instrumental in initiating the hormonal cascade of labor. The baby effectively begins the labor process when he or she is ready, and the hormonal (and energetic) dance of labor sets the stage for the initial experience of embodiment, the breastfeeding relationship, and the mother-child bond. Though there are many physiological benefits of natural birth, remembering the baby's participation in birth can be helpful when interventions are necessary.

Since a planned cesarean typically occurs before labor is initiated, speaking to the baby in a gentle manner about the approaching cesarean and "birth day" will engage the baby's energy in the process. I encourage mothers to tell their babies what is happening as any intervention occurs and to emphasize the joy of being able to see one another very soon. This can allay some of the fear around the medical process. A woman, or those assisting her, can bless the room and work with the birth energy to support any intervention or a cesarean birth. Likewise, she can work with the birth flow and connect to her baby energetically when intervention is necessary or even a transfer to a neonatal intensive care unit is required.

In the vulnerability and energetic openness of birthing, unplanned interventions can leave a strong imprint that overlays the whole birth experience. Again, the great learning for me has been that we can call forth the birth energy by working with a mother's body at any time, even thirty or forty years after her child is born. Likewise, by restoring the birth energy flow, such as with a simple energy meditation (page 116), the birth field and its meaning for mother and child can be cleared of the trauma imprint and restored to its radiant form. Though we would like to avoid trauma, repairing the energy connection affected by trauma makes potent medicine for navigating life's currents.

A Perspective of Trauma

As a pelvic care specialist, I have witnessed many varied aspects of pelvic trauma, including past physical or sexual abuse; medical procedures to the pelvis (particularly those done at an early age); gender wounds that formed when a child was unwanted because of her gender; and the profound loss from abortion, birth loss, loss of a family member, or even the stress of a contentious divorce. Because the pelvic bowl contains the root chakra—our sense of safety and security—it registers the impacts of these traumas. Even a job transfer, move, or change to the home or family can place added stress on the root.

The long-term effects of these stresses depend on the resources a woman has to counteract them. If she was a child when a trauma occurred, then the imprint will be more impactful. If she had parents or others who supported her through the trauma, or if she herself gained coping skills as an adult, then she will recover more fully. Pelvic trauma disrupts the alignment and flow of the pelvic energy, and though many people live with unresolved trauma, the impacts of trauma can be healed.

In fact, I began writing *Wild Feminine* in 2001 as a healing resource after witnessing my clients' pelvic trauma response to September 11. The day after September 11, in my Oregon-based women's health practice, I saw client after client who had a multitude of pelvic trigger points, high tension in the pelvic floor, and an energy pattern of dissonance that I find associated with a pelvic trauma response. None of the women had known anyone directly affected by September 11, yet their bodies were registering the disruption caused by this collective trauma.

With each of these clients, I worked with the tension patterns and alignment of energy in the pelvic bowl to restore a sense of peace in the center. This realignment is a way of resolving the impact caused by trauma. We are not always able to control the events of life; traumatic events occur, but we can minimize the imprint they make on our bodies and energy fields by restoring physical and energetic alignment in the core.

I witnessed the trauma imprints of September 11 as they were happening. However, most trauma patterns are carried from the past as less visible imprints, subtle tensions, and energy restrictions. If unaddressed, they affect our well-being, ability to connect with others, and access to our own creative abundance.

When Birth Stimulates Prior Trauma or Causes an Overwhelming Emotional Reaction

Birth events can be traumatic, and previous trauma can be restimulated by birthing. Past experiences of sexual or physical abuse or anything that threatened your sense of safety can be retriggered by the intensity of birth or the pelvic stimulation that birthing entails.

If after giving birth you find yourself overwhelmed and unable to find balance, then you may be in the midst of a trauma response or postpartum depression. If you are having difficulty taking care of yourself or your baby, feeling disoriented or agitated, or crying uncontrollably, these are signs that you are in a state of trauma or depression that requires professional assistance.

In the major transition that the postpartum period entails, you can experience emotional highs and lows. If these fluctuations in mood are extreme or you are unable to recover, seek professional counseling from a practitioner trained in trauma resolution and techniques for working with postpartum depression. Additional signs that indicate a trauma state also include a sense of bodily dis-connect, negative associations regarding the body, a sense of feeling incomplete, overwhelming feelings or repetitive thoughts, and dis-orientation or difficulty being present. If a woman had a traumatic birth herself, sometimes birthing can reactivate held trauma. For example, I have had clients who were adopted at birth and found that birthing brought up stored emotions of grief or loss.

Retriggered trauma and depression of any kind make it difficult to heal from birth while also addressing a newborn's high demands. However, the good news is that when the trauma arises it can also be addressed and resolved. With support from a skilled practitioner, you have the opportunity to heal the often inaccessible imprints of trauma or resolve the effects of depression so that they have less impact on your core sense of well-being. In addition to counseling, bodywork and acupuncture can restore the wholeness in your center. Baby bluesconnection.org is a good resource for mom-to-mom support.

Trauma disrupts the energy field; the bodily response to a trauma event alters the core energy like the rocks that rechannel the flow of a river. The key for working with any trauma, old or new, is to clear the trauma imprint, realign the energy field, and restore the energy flow. In the case of birth, we work with the actual birth field and birth energy flow. When we witness the disruptions caused by any trauma, we also witness the potential for resolution.

The Potency of the Birth Field and Energy Flow

Observing the birth field, I have come to understand the potency of this place as the connection point between spirit and body. We are meeting the divine within ourselves and receiving a limitless potential in this sacred transfer of birth energy. It shapes how we understand the world and ourselves as creative beings. Elena Tonetti, a Russian-born leader in the field of water birth, holds "birthshops," or workshops to assist adults in reimprinting their birth events. (To learn more, visit birthintobeing.com.) She has witnessed the potential within each participant to establish a new reference point in their nervous system, switching from an imprint of initial chaos or wounding to a new imprint of love and full support.

Likewise, we can reframe the birth field in our bodies regardless of our birthing experience and then access this new potential as mothers. When women enter my office carrying the imprint of a traumatic birth event, it creates a field of turbulence in their center and continues to disrupt the energy flow in their body well beyond the birth. Restoring the alignment of the birth field is like placing a radiant crystal back into their core body; it reshapes and energizes everything. In this process, we also imprint an ability to recover from difficult experiences. This means we can more readily access other healing fields by making ritual, visiting sacred sites and wild places, and engaging the creative energy that is meant to flow through and infuse our daily lives.

Women's Stories: Midwifing the Birth Energy

Maia came for pelvic work to address some physical effects of childbirth and a general sense of feeling disconnected from her body. She had planned for a home birth, and though she labored for two days at home, she ended up transporting to the hospital. The hospital staff was accommodating, and she labored on for many additional hours. But her labor stalled, and when her baby's heart rate began to drop, she eventually had a cesarean birth.

Though her child was now two years old, Maia continued to feel a sense of failure in regard to the birth. She had prepared herself diligently and could not understand why she was unable to have a vaginal birth. Maia had some mild incontinence (urine leakage) when she laughed or coughed and had difficulty engaging her pelvic muscles. Maia also felt no libido and cut off from her lower body ever since the birth, so she and her partner were rarely having sex.

Maia's sense of bodily disconnect could be partially an emotional response to a traumatic birth. But this sense of disconnection may have been compounded by the cesarean surgery; the horizontal incision can actually disrupt the energy or chi lines in the body. Natural birth can stretch pelvic muscles and affect their ability to engage—until a women receives vaginal massage to rebalance the tissues—but any added stress can accentuate these effects. Both the prolonged labor and stress of transporting from home to hospital likely added to Maia's pelvic strain and postpartum symptoms, which could have persisted for years without pelvic care. Many women are surprised to have pelvic symptoms with a cesarean, but the strain on the uterus and pelvic organs during surgery can also cause tension in the pelvic fascia.

It is common to have a dampened libido in the first year postpartum, due to hormones and the depletion that occurs with caring for a newborn. However, a complete lack of libido after birthing or a low libido that persists past the first year both suggest pelvic imbalances. In Maia's case, she had both physical imbalances and a disrupted birth flow that were impacting her pelvic connection and core energy—and likely affecting her libido as well.

For Maia's treatment, I began with internal massage to restore core alignment in the pelvic bowl. I noted the stagnation in her pelvic or root energy. Stagnation is a sense of energetic holding or congestion, like an overly full closet. I invited Maia to bring awareness to her pelvic bowl and breathe from her bowl downward, releasing the pent-up heat, which I encourage women to send downward into the earth. This heat is often palpable in the pelvis; a woman herself might notice the increased temperature in her lower body. With breath moving the energy downward, the heat dissipates.

As Maia released the excess energy from the birth field, I watched her relax into a new and radiant energy pattern. When alignment is restored in the field, the birth energy can flow. I suggested that she imagine her child as both the new-born and her present age of two. Maia imagined her daughter as both the baby on her belly and the toddler running around her, and then began to breathe the birth energy of her womb toward these images of her child. With cesarean birth, I sug-gest that women imagine the birth energy moving through the vagina and the cesarean scar, to complete the natural vagi-nal flow and to honor the baby's physical birth. Maia's pelvis released more heat, and I sensed the movement of her child's essence releasing into the birth field like water rippling out when a pebble touches its surface.

When I lead this exercise with a woman while her baby is in the room, as soon as the birth energy flows, the baby often responds by moving and vocalizing. Twice I have seen a baby begin to turn their body, as if traveling down the birth canal, in response to the birth energy coming into the room. In both of these cases, the babies were having difficulty nursing. After seeing their response to the release of the birth energy, we brought each baby to the mother's breast, and each latched more fully and vigorously. This energetic thread between mother and baby, and the fact that we can access this ancient energy bond for healing, is profound and hardly understood.

Though Maia's daughter was no longer a newborn, she would still feel the rebalancing in the birth energy. As Maia's energy. Immediately, tears filled her eyes. I asked if she wanted to restore a sense of peace in the birth field by doing an energy meditation, and she nodded silently.

I suggested that Maia return to the last time she felt a good connection to her body while birthing. She relayed that it was when she was still pregnant and laboring at home. I invited her to begin her visualization there, at home. When a women realigns her birth field, she can be anywhere she chooses. The physical aspect of birth has been completed at a discrete point, but the energy is more fluid and can travel across space and time and has vital information for mothering.

In these birth energy meditations, I act as an energetic midwife, holding space for a woman while she clears any imprint of trauma and aligns with the original potential of the birthing field. In Maia's case, the birth field imprinted the trauma of the transport and cesarean and interrupted her ability to integrate the birth experience. Connecting with her body was difficult because each time she did so it reminded her of the traumatic aspects of the birth, filling her with remorse and self-doubt.

However, we can return to this birth field to clear the trauma and realign the overall energy. This process can resolve the imprints of a difficult birth and restore a woman's pure connection to her body and baby. I have developed these skills for working with the birth field from my understanding of the energy of the pelvic bowl and through assisting many women in recovering their rightful birth energy flow.

With Maia, I led her through the birth energy meditations shared in the next section. As she visualized herself birthing at home, I invited her to release any energy from the hospital or surgery or any other difficult aspects of the birth. Releasing the trauma imprint from the birth field is like clearing turbulent or disorganized energy. At first there is a swirling center came into contact with the peaceful radiance of the birth field, she remarked how much better she felt. When the birth field is out of balance, a woman often feels unbalanced herself. Restoring alignment in the core of the body and the birth field is essential for living and mothering from that place. When Maia left my office, she looked completely different. Her color was robust and she exuded a happy glow.

Maia returned two weeks later to share how everything had shifted. Maia herself felt whole again and more inclined to find connection with her partner. She had a renewed and empowered connection to her body, recognizing that it was not only her place to birth from but also to mother from. The physical work had resolved many of her pelvic symptoms, and she felt the first impulses of her libido returning.

Feeling reconnected to her body made Maia's days easier. Gone was the sense of struggle that she thought was simply a part of parenting. Maia's daughter had been noticeably calmer and more secure, with less frequent night awakenings and fewer tantrums. Maia continued the birth energy meditation at home. One night, as they lay together, Maia spoke with her daughter about their hard work during the birth and that she had some new birth energy to give to her. Maia then breathed this birth energy to her daughter, who laughed and clapped her hands as if receiving a present. From many of the mothers I have worked with, I have heard similar reports, either of a profound experience of reconnecting and a tangible change in a child or the mother-child bond. The children seem to have more capacity themselves and are able to sense more and draw upon the strength of their bond from the restored birth energy flow. This is the potential of our amazing female bodies that not only gestate but contain the essence of life.

The Birth Energy Flow Connects Mother and Child

Clearing trauma from the birth field means that a woman is able to restore and then access the birth energy flow, strengthening the connection between herself and her child. I explain to mothers that birth is not a separation, where we lose the close internal bond with our child, nor is it like holding on to their energy as if it were a kite string. Instead, the birth energy flows like a river through a woman's body to her child for all time.

In a child's early years, the birth energy flow is coupled with the intensive physical connection of holding, nursing, and caring for a child. But as children grow, they move further into the world, and this bond becomes less physical and more energetic. Wherever we are in our mothering journey, we can continue to give our children a strong energy current by focusing on the river of energy between us. We may send this birth energy in meditation, with a touch or quiet nod, to soothe a frustration or infuse their life with blessing in any moment.

When one of my sons prepared for a fifth-grade overnight trip, we discussed the approaching separation. I have noticed that parenting with connection, such as bed sharing, baby wearing, and prolonged nursing, makes for children who are not only secure but also more content to be in the home. The thought of a night away may stretch their comfort level.

I invited my son to close his eyes and feel the river of energy running between us. "Can you feel it?" I asked him.

"Yes!" was his enthusiastic response. I told him to sense into this connection whenever he missed home, because it was always there to support him.

The thread of life between you and your child can be a source of sustenance for both of you as your child moves further into the world. The child can receive this potential, and you can give support by sending an offering of energy to them from this place.

There are many worries as a parent. Whenever a worry arises, try sending your child a blessing along this birth flow. Worry tends to contract and restrict energy, while blessings align and enhance its flow. In fact, a mother's worry about her child may cause her to unintentionally hold on to the birth energy in an attempt to hold back and "protect" her child. However, we cannot keep them from their lives. Worry will not make them safe. Our best protection is our presence, and the power of the blessing energy from the spirit door. Sending a blessing can counter the effects of worry and bring helpful energies to any situation. We can also energize this connection with intentional bursts of love for our children and all children; they are the future, and the birth energy blesses their way.

In mothering three children and working as a healer, I am more aware than ever how sensitive our babies and children are to the trauma or disruptions that may occur for them. In the face of this sensitivity, the feeling of responsibility can be paralyzing, lest a mother ever make a misstep in pregnancy, birth, or mothering that wounds her child. I want all mothers to know that along with this responsibility also comes abundant medicine and creative vitality, and we can find our inherent healing potential if we go to the center of ourselves. How you birth does not define your mothering.

If there is a separation at birth from a trauma or even adoption, connecting to the birth flow, from womb to child, can assist the repair. I have worked with women whose children were taken for resuscitation at birth. These mothers can feel a sense of separation from their child or a sense of chaos in the bond as a result of the early trauma imprint. I guide them through a birth flow meditation where they return, in their mind's eye, to the moment just before the child's birth. Then we sweep the trauma imprint away as if sweeping dust with a broom, seeing or sensing this energy moving down into the earth. After moving the trauma energy out of the birth field, they visualize the birth flow reconnecting them with their child. After the session, I encourage them to send this birth energy as a blessing, in their mind's eye, whenever they need assistance with this child or simply want to strengthen their bond. It is a powerful way for resetting this energy connection (see the Women's Stories on page 269).

If a woman has more than one child or even twins, she may notice a challenge in connecting with the one who had a difficult birth or required medical assistance. As soon as she clarifies the birth field and repairs any energetic disruptions, these imbalances shift. The ease in her mother-child relationships will reflect this new potential. A mother can also tap into this birth flow to reinforce a positive connection with her child in any moment or with any challenge.

If you have any imprint of disruption at birth, you can do the following exercises for realigning the birth field and restoring the birth energy flow in order to correct these energetic effects. The birth energy can be realigned regardless of the circumstances of the birth event or present age of your child. You may do the exercises on your own or in the presence of your child. Then observe the changes in yourself and your child. Allow your feelings to arise or tears to flow. Rather than framing birth into a "good" or "bad" experience, understand that each one assists your learning and growth. Once you heal the birth energy connection, use this meditation on a routine basis as one of your mothering tools.

Note: You may do the following meditation in order to set up an energetic birth field for a child who has been adopted or to send blessings to a child you gave up for adoption.

Exercise: Realigning the Birth Field

1. For this meditation, prepare a quiet space where you will be undisturbed. Reflect upon the experience and the energy of your birth event. Sense the quality of energy from the birth

field by pondering the birth. How does it feel? What do you notice? Are there any densities or contracted aspects? Remain neutral and simply observe with compassion.

2. Now engage the energy by sensing and seeing it with your inner eye. If there are aspects of fear or trauma, sweep them away as if sweeping the floor. Let any difficulties dissipate. See these imprints as dust or matter, and move them toward the earth with each sweep. If there were any disruptive people or practitioners at the birth, sweep their negative energy away. Clear any remorse, guilt, or grief as well. Restore the connection with your body; remember that your body birthed as best it was able. You need this beautiful body to mother your child; reclaim the potential of your creative center. Continue until the birth field is clear and filled with radiant light or a sense of ease.

3. When the field is clear, return to the last moment you felt connected to the birth flow. Imagine yourself there in a safe and peaceful place, with the people whose presence you desire. Notice how it feels to be in your desired place; sink into the sensations of ease and comfort (all difficulty is over).

4. Begin to bless the birth field. Imagine a golden light moving in the air around you, bringing a divine energy that ignites the life force in all that it touches. See the space around your body responding to this light. Notice how it feels. Breathe toward the sacred energy of your birth field as it realigns. With your inner vision or senses, witness the pattern that emerges as the spirit door opens and receive its blessing.

5. Continue with the next exercise, Restoring the Birth Energy Flow and Bond.

Exercise: Restoring the Birth Energy Flow and Bond

1. As the birth field realigns, now you may restore the birth energy flow and receive a new imprint.

2. Begin by sensing your child in the womb; see him or her in your mind's eye and feel their energy. (Even if your child is adopted, sense him or her in the same way.) Remember your child's earliest beginning, held in the womb space. Also imagine your child as his or her present age, not in the womb but in the space around you. Let the energy between you both connect and align.

3. If your baby was separated from you at birth due to any intervention or trauma, sweep away all the trauma or interference energy and observe it dissipating or moving into the earth. In your mind's eye, bring your baby back to your chest. Connect the birth flow from womb to chest.

4. Now begin to breathe the energy through the spirit door, from your womb to your child. (If he or she is adopted, receive the energy for this child from the birth mother and give thanks for her sharing of this thread.) Continue to breathe the energy down through your womb and vagina (or cesarean incision), toward your baby. Sense the soul essence of your child moving through your center. See the energy moving like a river of light through your body, touching your chest where your child would initially lie in the first moments after birth and then outward to him or her at their present age. This river has no end; you are simply opening this current of life. Once it is flowing strongly, see the energy moving through your body and the birth field to your child,

at present age, and filling his or her energy field. This is the life force that informs their essence and their journey, as well as your journey together. Witness the miracle of this light.

5. As the birth energy flows, notice your own energy field. Are you receiving the blessing of this energy? Let go of any hesitations you might have to accept this path or become a mother. To inhabit your full mothering and creative potential, you must step fully through the spirit door with your child's entry. Let the birth energy assist you; it contains infinite resources for making an inspired mothering pattern when you release yourself into the flow. This energy can also assist the family in realigning; let this birth energy radiate into the whole family energy field. You may talk to your child, sharing your original desires for their birth and how the birth energy now contains a blessing for them.

6. Make an intention for your mothering and set it in this sacred birth space. Let the light of the spirit door reveal your next form. Always remember the potent medicine here; call upon this birth flow for inspiration and energy along the way.

Healing the Womb: Miscarriage and Other Pregnancy Losses

When a child is carried full-term, the birth flow becomes part of his or her life force and guides a mother's care. If a pregnancy begins but does not complete its gestation, there is still a river of energy between a woman and her child's spirit, though it has a more ethereal quality.

I learned about the post-miscarriage energy flow to a child's spirit from my own miscarriage. By honing my energy skills in my work with women, I had a greater ability to sense it. Perhaps the people living close to the earth and practicing more ancient forms of medicine recognize these womb connections to spirit. We could do more to support women in reconnecting to their bodies and the potency that resides there to assist their recovery from a birth loss.

Early miscarriages happen frequently but can cause a profound sense of loss. This is particularly the case when they occur in succession or without a subsequent full-term pregnancy. Though a pregnancy does not replace the loss, there is some resolution when a baby completes a full gestation in the womb.

Miscarriage as a first birthing event can also be physically painful, since the womb must contract and open more widely for the miscarriage than it does for menstruation. My own miscarriage came after a full-term labor and delivery, and as a result, was a gentle experience. But for many women who have a miscarriage, it is a painful and confusing event because they typically have the miscarriage on their own without labor support. It's important to seek direct support from a medical provider during a miscarriage.

Ectopic pregnancy can be traumatic not only for the loss but for any potential rupture or surgery that may accompany the loss because it is a medical emergency. This progression is so rapid that the pace of the pregnancy and loss is a profound shock to the body. In contrast, late-term and full-term loss, occurring after a woman has held the baby in her womb for an extended time, leaves a deep imprint of grief in the center of her being.

Though each of these losses will leave women mourning, there is also a blessing that can be received with such intimate womb encounters. I have sat at the spirit door while working with these women, and we have both been affected by the baby spirits who have come in to these sessions. These experiences have only deepened my awe for the doorway that lies in the female body and for the spirits who may visit us there.

I include an exercise here for reconnecting with a baby spirit and restoring the energy current. This is the same exercise I use in my work. However, this meditation is only a small component of an integrated framework that can include grief counseling, bodywork, acupuncture, and other resources as needed. Healing in the face of great loss requires collective support from skilled practitioners.

Remember that miscarriage and other losses are birth events that require physical and energetic recovery. Traveling to the spirit door is a sacred experience that requires the same postpartum rest and nourishment to process all that has occurred. After my own miscarriage, I experienced a three-month period of a new inner space and quiet that initiated a major transformation.

Exercise: Energy Medicine for Pregnancy Loss

1. First prepare a space for this meditation in a quiet place where you will be undisturbed.

2. Bring attention to your womb, the place that held your baby. Sense your connection to this baby spirit. In loss, this connection is often there, deep within the womb. Go to your center and find your baby's spirit.

3. Talk with your baby. Ask how you might honor or remember him or her. Let your tears or grief move toward the earth.

4. After you have reconnected with your baby's spirit, breathe the thread of connection from your womb and out into your energy field. You will have more access to the essence of this spirit connection once you let the energy flow. Though you have experienced a loss, this energy thread is always here for receiving the blessings of this spirit child.

5. Whenever the grief of your loss arises, imagine yourself held by the Great Mother or ancient energy of the earth. There is always a presence that will hold us if we let ourselves be held. If it is warm, lie upon the earth and set your weariness down. It is in the surrender that new life and new hope can take hold again. *May spirit light your way.*

Reframing Your Birth Imprint for Mothering

Birth is one snapshot, but your mothering imprint is decades long. Though mothering is influenced by the birth, it is more profoundly shaped by your lifelong relationship with your child. By recalling the joyful aspects of a birth, you reinforce these imprints as support for your mothering. In pondering the birth, you may notice themes or opportunities for new potential within the layers of the experience. Additionally, by examining any losses in the birth field or flow, you can reframe this initial imprint. For example, if you did not receive enough support during the birth, be sure to create support for yourself in the postpartum and mothering time. Heal this imprint and therefore be able to receive support as a mother. If not addressed directly, challenging aspects of birth may affect the postpartum period or unconsciously influence your mothering. When challenging aspects are identified, they can be resolved by restoring the necessary energy flow and taking healing actions.

Prior to having a second pregnancy and birth event, or even to integrate the experience of a previous birth, I recommend completing a birth-review exercise like the one that follows. Reviewing your birth event completes a creative cycle, expands your perspective and resources, and enables your recovery from a challenging birth or a miscarriage. Conceiving a child after a miscarriage can bring up fear of another loss. In my second pregnancy, after a miscarriage, I had to consciously move through fear to connect with the baby in my womb. Engaging what is held in your body in relationship to past birth events is part of preparing and recovering; it gives you access to the deep energy currents of spirit and provides a salve for any fear or anxiety that may arise in the transformative process that occurs with every pregnancy. Restoring the full creative capacity in your center allows you to savor and bear witness in these journeys to the spirit door.

Reviewing Your Birth Event

Just as there is magic in conceiving and birthing a child, there is an ongoing mystery in engaging the birth field even long after giving birth. Take time to review your birth event. Ponder any areas of disruption in order to restore the energy flow. Recall the blessings, lessons, and energy potentials that arose. Share your birth story and the new patterns that emerged by writing it out or telling it to at least one other person. The following reflections may offer guidance:

When was the birth energy flowing strongly and the birth field aligned?

Are there any disruptions that need to be addressed?

What moments stand out to you in the birthing process? What gems do they contain?

What aspects of your birth event are cause for celebration? How do they assist your mothering?

What did you learn from this birth? How will this knowledge influence you?

Is there any grief in this birth event? How would you like to engage or move this grief?

If the birth feels incomplete or was difficult, do the exercises for realigning the birth field and restoring the birth energy flow. Then make note of what changes. What did you learn?

A Story of Three Generations:
Healing Birth across Time

I was walking with a friend in the park one day. She had given birth to her daughter nearly thirty years earlier and was lamenting her birthing experience. Her daughter had recently said that she was preparing for her first pregnancy, which prompted my friend to share her difficult birth story with me. The trauma had never been addressed and continued to have a profound imprint on her life.

As we walked, my friend relayed her story of a natural birth that was initially progressing well. She was almost completely dilated and near transition when a nurse recommended using a scalp probe to check the baby's response to the contractions (a procedure where a probe is inserted into the baby's scalp, now rarely performed except in high-risk pregnancies). The doctor asked his intern to conduct the test and departed, saying that my friend would be ready to push when he returned. In between powerful contractions, she had to recline so the intern could insert the scalp probe, but he was unsuccessful the first few times. Her baby started to react and pull back from the pelvic engagement, moving herself away from the sharp sensation at her crown.

My friend said that the birth never felt right from that moment on. She continued to labor, but her baby was no longer fully engaged in the pelvis. The baby's up-and-down movement caused a lip of the cervix to swell. The birth ended with a cesarean. My friend mourned the disruption that had occurred and the incomplete sensation from not pushing her baby out. Worse yet, when she was being stitched up from the cesarean, the anesthesiologist unknowingly gave her too high a dose of a sedative, and she was unable to stay awake for the bonding time after the birth, which was very important to her.

Hearing her story while walking through the park, I suggested that we change this three-decade-long imprint with an energy meditation. I invited her to choose one of the trees along the path and to sit against the tree's trunk. She chose a large sycamore tree, sat down at its base, and closed her eyes. She called to mind the birth of her daughter, and the air around her took on a contracted and chaotic energy—the trauma imprint in the birth field.

I led her through the birth field realignment and birth flow meditations (page 116), inviting her to move the interference energy out of the birth field. What began as a contracted birth field shifted to become spacious and calm. The air spun gently around her, reminding me of birth movements that occur as a baby turns and moves down through the pelvis, while she began to breathe the birth energy from her womb toward her now-grown daughter. Tears flowed and the light changed as the birth energy was restored.

We continued until the meditation felt complete. Though it was a simple process, the effects were palpable. My friend was more grounded and her energy was bright, though she would shed more tears as the birth flow continued. Later she shared that her daughter had called while we were working. (As I mentioned, children of all ages feel the movement of birth energy as it realigns.)

Her daughter had phoned from the land she and her partner were planning to purchase, to say that she had been lying on a bridge on the land and meditating, thinking of the love in her family and hoping that their offer would be accepted. Later that day they found out that they would be the farm's new owners. That night they conceived their son. As her daughter said, "Good morphic field energy that day!" Or perhaps good birth flow energy in a newly aligned birth field. When my friend visited her daughter's new property a week later, she was amazed to see a giant sycamore tree in the center of the yard, just like the one she had sat beneath for the birth meditation.

Less than nine months later, her daughter gave birth at home, on this land, to my friend's grandchild. At a point in the birth when the dilation was almost but not quite complete, both my friend and her daughter felt momentarily discouraged. Then my friend called to mind the new birth pattern made while sitting under the sycamore tree that day. She brought this expanded potential into the birth of her grandchild, and the birth energy began to move.

My friend held her daughter while her daughter pushed her baby out. Holding her daughter in this way, she had a sense of the pushing in her own body and a completion previously unrealized in her own birthing experience. From mother to daughter to grandchild, a healing of birth energy passed down the lineage line.

SIX

Caretaking the Mothering Body and Soul

Mothering invites us back to the center, and in order to caretake the body and soul of our mothering, we must shift any habit or structure that beckons us away from this center point. Mothers know intimately the challenge of the modern divide between work or professional life and home life. They frequently experience isolation or a loss in identity, the challenge of leaving young children in order to work, and the difficulty of making an income because of this work-home separation. However, this divide has a greater cost to the entire community; our energetic reserves are depleted when the home fires remain untended. The soul hungers for our creative presence in the home and other inner realms. The call back to the center of our bodies in mothering also invites a whole new manner of living.

Creating a New Way to Work

To make a living and a flexible schedule, I found that after having my children, I was actually much better prepared to create something on my own rather than work for someone else. In developing my own business, there was more work to do outside regular hours, but there was also tremendous flexibility in my work schedule that could accommodate our family needs.

My first son was one year old when I started my private women's health practice. I rented an affordable office and worked two partial days. When he was sick, I could easily reschedule my clients for another day. With my second newborn, I left work for three months and then resumed a schedule that evolved with my son's breastfeeding. As he transitioned to solid food, I gradually added time to my workdays until I was working three-quarter days and then two full days. I repeated this process with my third child, and over time I have tailored my work schedule around my family life.

Being a woman who loves both her children and her work, I believe that women can more readily create what they want for themselves by applying their creativity to the task. It also helps to know that your baby or child's needs will change over time. For example, though I began working in my private practice when my children were three months old, I set up a brief working schedule in this early period. I also kept each postpartum year free of major commitments, such as travel or workshops, so that the overall load on me was as light as possible, making space for the main work of integrating my new baby while restoring my post-birth body. As my children have grown, my work schedule has evolved as well.

Whether rebalancing work and home, reconnecting with your partner, or creating ways of mothering that sustain you, be patient with this phase of learning and developing new structures for your life. It takes time to establish new patterns of energy flow and rebuild your framework for mothering.

Connecting with Touch and
Tending the Home Fire

My intention in scheduling my work life around my children was so that we could be in contact—literally be able to touch one another. In the first year, I felt as if something was missing from my own body when I was away from my child longer than about four hours. They often became distraught as well when we were separated for longer. We needed one another; our bodies and energy systems complemented one another. Being in close contact is essential in establishing the mother-child bond. Finding a way to be in close contact may require some changes to the patterns around the home that were established prior to having a child.

In the bodies of the children I work with, there is a greater suppleness in the ones who are frequently touched and more tension in those for whom touching is less a part of their routine. For my own children, I have noticed that simply being held in my arms is relaxing for them. They like to be held or stay close beside me, even as they have become older. Our mothering bodies naturally align and energize our children's bodies, just with our presence and our touch.

Touch is also an essential component of healing and restored vitality. When one of my children is sick, I clear space to be with him. When they were still taking naps, I often slept with them and remained nearby until they awoke. They seek the comfort of our continuous presence and being in the home. Though tending the home fire is not typically valued in the external or professional world, as an energy reader, I recognize how precious it is for banking deep stores of energy.

The home fire is where each of us draws our life-giving nourishment, whether by resting, eating, spending time with a partner, or raising a family. Working in the yard, making food, and cleaning or organizing are all ways of regenerating the home energy. Picking my son up from preschool one day, he asked if I was working at home while he was gone (as opposed to going to my office). I told him I was indeed doing work at home, to which he responded by kissing my hand in an enthusiastic flurry. Hearing that I was home, even while he was not, made him happy. Children intuitively know the value of being in the home; tending the home builds our energetic wealth. I have nursed, carried, co-slept, and cherished the bodies of each one of my children. In doing so I have come home to my own body, to my creative center, and literally to my home.

In the early days of living in our house, before children, my husband and I had our first baby in the form of a gorgeous female German shepherd, Kiva. We hired a dog sitter for her because we spent long workdays away from the home. Giving birth to our first child was an initiation back into the home. I left my formal job, and my husband's environmental organization suggested he work from home when their downtown office was relocated. We came home and never left. Kiva thrived with the new arrangement, and so did we.

Work life is not always so flexible and may require that a mother leave the home even while her child is young. Women can use their creative potential to examine their options. Some couples make a schedule where they trade off being at home to share the home-based caretaking. Perhaps a schedule can be reduced or altered during the first six months to a year of a child's life. Coming up with alternative ways of doing work is an option. Though I had few work models beyond hospital or clinic-based physical therapy, I chose to open my own small practice, with a low overhead. It was successful, and I set my own hours.

Additionally, reconnecting with touch is beneficial when a mother is away for an extended period. She can return home and increase mother-child contact by wearing her baby in a sling or snuggling with her child while reading a book together. Co-sleeping is a particularly important opportunity to catch up on time together.

Touch restores the energy flow and the bond between you, and helps you both clear pent-up stress.

Even as children become older, they benefit from touch as a way to stay present in their bodies. When children are touched, they more readily contact their own center and are able to receive the wisdom it contains, which may run counter to the information from the outer world. Touch from a thoughtful parent or caretaker is calming and helps release the stresses or emotional energies that arise in navigating relationships and the ups and downs of life. No matter the age or gender of your child, he or she needs your touch. Sustain a practice in your family of exchanging shoulder or foot massages and giving regular hugs—making touch a part of parenting throughout your child's life. Even with a simple touch to your child, notice how your energy aligns with one another and reaffirms a centered presence of being together.

Birth and then mothering will initiate a thousand new ways of being in your own body and as a mother-child pair. Let this initiation move you away from a life that is likely weighted toward the exterior, and back toward your own center and the creative essence that arises from within.

What initiation are you receiving presently?
How are you being called to tend the home fire?
What new forms are arising in your life?

. . . .

DROPPING PERFECTION AND BEING THE GOOD-ENOUGH MOTHER

If we perceive mothering as a journey rather than a destination, then we can also see it as an opportunity to learn and transform. We are not meant to be perfect; we are meant to expand what we know. We may have challenges or work schedules that remain outside our control, yet we can be present with the needs that arise in ourselves or in our children as a result.

Perfection is a narrow pathway and a rigid one prone to shattering. Being a good-enough mother means that you bring your vibrant self to the equation but in a manner that allows you to evolve and grow. Be open to insights and inspiration and even to your child's own skills rising up to meet you. In mothering from the center, the child you are tending will also grow and change in his or her capacity. Being good enough, rather than perfect, means there is room for whatever life and spirit bring.

....

The Future of Postpartum Care

To encourage the caretaking of our feminine selves and center point for our mothering, I am igniting a healthcare movement to provide better care for the postpartum body. The current emphasis is on caring for our body during pregnancy, with virtually nothing to address the myriad of birthing effects or postpartum needs. The primary focus of my women's health practice and teaching program for healthcare providers is based on holistic and physical/energetic medicine for the pelvic bowl. This physical and energetic medicine is vital women's pelvic care and absolutely essential postpartum—yet it is hardly known. In France, however, women receive ten to twenty government-sponsored sessions of physical therapy for the pelvic floor as *routine postnatal care*—a cultural recognition of the importance of root health for women. The next feminist movement: government-sponsored care of the pelvic bowl as a measure of overall progress for women.

As mothers who do a tremendous amount for our families, our bodies deserve quality care. Even though I am a women's health physical therapist, it was years before I thought to apply pelvic care to my own body as pregnancy preparation. The current model of care is to treat pelvic symptoms rather than address pelvic imbalance by way of preventative medicine. In my work at a local hospital earlier in my career, most of my clients were in their sixties and seventies. By the chronic nature of their pelvic patterns, I recognized that they had been living with pelvic imbalances for twenty, thirty, or more years. I wondered why we were not addressing women's pelvic health in a more holistic manner.

Having a baby initiates a profound bodily transformation and is an invitation to embody a new potential. The changes in your body from birthing and the demands of nursing and tending your child may at times be overwhelming, but recognize that you are being remade and finding a new form. When your child requests to nurse, touch, or be held, embrace these reminders that the essence of life exists most potently in the now. Your child invites you to be more present and fully embodied in your own center. Call upon the healers in your community to restore your postpartum body to radiance.

Understanding Pelvic Imbalances

The primary mode of addressing pelvic imbalances, besides surgery, is to suggest that a woman do Kegels, or exercises that squeeze the pelvic muscles to strengthen them. However, most pelvic imbalances are not caused by weakness and will not change with a Kegel exercise. The majority of pelvic issues are the result of imbalances in the muscle recruitment pattern, diminished elasticity in the fascia or muscle fibers, inhibition of the muscles, and poor organ position. These issues are directly addressed only with vaginal massage, a pelvic care technique that restores core muscle, organ, and fascial balance in the pelvic bowl so that the muscles function in a dynamic and balanced manner. Additionally, imbalances in the root energy must be addressed to recover core vibrance as well.

After I gave birth to my first son, I experienced pelvic pain from scar tissue that formed in response to receiving a few stitches to address a minor tear from the birth. My vagina became irritated, and sex was painful. Yet I was busy learning how to attend to my newborn and paid little attention to my own body.

Several months passed, and sex only became more painful. At about six months postpartum, I sought care from one of my women's health mentors, and she did a session of internal vaginal massage. Though I required nine additional months of vaginal self-massage to be pain free, the one session made a marked difference in reducing my pain and increasing my comfort. I had been living with a tremendous knot of tension in my pelvic muscles from the physical impact of birth and the pelvic irritation caused by the stitches. The session released most of the tension, and I felt a new sense of blood flow and vibrance in my center.

Receiving vaginal massage to support my own recovery from birthing was transformative. I was inspired to start a women's health practice with a holistic focus. For more than a decade now, I have been addressing women's pelvic health in a more preventative and holistic manner. My women's practice now includes women at all stages of life. I have seen the benefits of addressing pelvic imbalances directly after birthing, as pregnancy prevention, or general women's wellness. Any woman experiencing post-birth pelvic symptoms is given a priority to be seen because I know that with one visit I can greatly enhance her sense of well-being.

A mother traveled from California to see me for postpartum pelvic care. An avid hiker before childbirth, she suffered from pelvic symptoms that prevented her from even walking a block. In a single session, we restored pelvic muscle balance and set her body in the proper stage for healing. A month later, I received a photo of her backpacking with her daughter, a broad smile on her face. If a mother feels right in her root, everything else she does flows from there.

How to Find Healing for the Vagina and Pelvis

Being a pelvic floor therapist, I want women to have more information about the potential postpartum changes in the pelvic bowl as well as the ways to find healing. Birth is a normal process for our bodies. However, each birth is different, and a woman can experience a range of postpartum effects on the vagina and pelvis from pregnancy and birth.

To accommodate a growing baby and allow for the birth, the abdominal and pelvic region must stretch tremendously. A cesarean birth still produces strain on the pelvic core, both from the surgery and the force required to lift the baby from the uterus. Also, because we are increasingly sedentary in our jobs and lives, the pelvic muscles are more congested and less dynamic, even before pregnancy. We need ways to reduce congestion and restore pelvic health both to enhance core vitality and to heal from the birth process.

A Range of Postpartum Effects

After a birth experience, a woman's vagina is often swollen and a little numb. She may feel a heaviness from the stretch in the vaginal walls, which can make walking quite uncomfortable. She may scarcely be able to engage her abdominal or pelvic muscles in their post-birth stretched position. Urination is often slow, and a woman's tissues are sensitive. Any scar tissue from post-birth stitches may irritate her vaginal tissues. Again, most women hardly know that there is a profession that can assist their recovery because most women's health physical therapy is utilized at menopause or beyond and typically with more severe symptoms.

Healing my postpartum body with the internal massage techniques from my women's health training was empowering and sparked a dialogue with my own center. Not only did this pelvic connection and self-care ease my mind for subsequent births, but I actually had less tearing and more resilience in my vaginal tissues, even as I birthed additional children. With my first birth, I used massage to stretch my perineum in the weeks before my son's labor, but I did so with a mechanical approach rather than one of connection with my own body. It was caretaking my pelvic bowl on a routine basis that increased my pelvic resilience for birthing.

Paying attention to their body after birthing, women do notice the changes in their vagina, in regard to sensation or appearance, from the stretch in the vaginal tissues. Any intervention such as forceps, episiotomy, catheter, or stitching—though possibly necessary—may add to the feeling of disruption or stretch in the vaginal tissues. In major tears, stitch repairs done by a skilled surgeon can greatly assist overall healing and actually prevent long-term pelvic issues. And some of the stretch and swelling in the vagina and pelvis will resolve on their own with time. But many of the changes continue to have effects on a more subtle level unless a woman receives assistance from a women's health physical therapist, a Holistic Pelvic Care therapist (see wildfeminine.com for a list), or another practitioner skilled in physical medicine techniques for restoring alignment in the core. In fact, these techniques ought to be a part of our practice of annual women's healthcare and self-care to address pelvic symptoms preventatively, restore the flow of creative energy, prevent long-term issues, and enhance core vitality.

Exercise: Basic Pelvic Anatomy and Energetics

In my women's health practice, I find that very few women know the anatomy of the pelvic bowl. It is easier to care for something that is known, so I teach basic pelvic anatomy and energy as part of a woman's self-care. Do the following exercise to learn the land marks of your own pelvic bowl and feel the grounding energy of your core.

1. First locate the landmarks of your pelvis on your body. Place your hands on the upper boundary of your pelvic bowl (the pelvic crest), sometimes referred to incorrectly as your hips. Move your hands to the front of your pelvis to find your pubic bone. This is your pubic symphysis where the two halves of the pelvis meet. Then slide your hands toward the back of the pelvis. Here the pelvic bones connect with the sacrum, a beautiful triangle-shaped bone. Sense into the vibrancy of your pelvic bones, this boundary for your pelvic bowl.

2. Close your eyes and imagine your pelvic bowl. Sense the spaciousness within your bowl and notice your inner awareness of this space. You may feel a boundary marked by the bones of your pelvis, but the energy of the bowl is broader than this boundary. Trace the bony boundaries of your pelvis and again sense both the physical and energetic shape of your pelvic bowl.

3. Bring awareness to your womb, the deep center of your pelvic bowl. Notice the creative well in your core. Connect with this place that holds your children and serves as the doorway for their essence as well as any other heartfelt creations.

4. Sense the ovaries on either side of the womb, the creative radiance that lights each side of your bowl. The left ovary is related to your feminine fire and the source of your inspiration. The

right ovary is related to your masculine fire and the form that you find for creative expression. Notice whether these fires are bright or are in need of tending.

5. At the base of your inner pelvis is your pelvic floor. The pelvic floor relates to the root chakra, an energetic place that imprints your sense of safety, belonging, and earth connection. The energy here determines your ability to embody your creative capacity or give form to spirit.

6. In the center of the pelvic floor is your vaginal opening and passageway. The lovemaking you receive, the blood of your cycle, and any babies you birth vaginally all pass through this gateway. Even with cesarean births, energy releases from the vagina and can be consciously accessed by breathing and visualizing the birth energy moving through the root. What is your connection with this precious gateway, this guardian of your root? What are you presently releasing or bringing in for your creative core?

7. The pelvic bowl holds your creative essence, the gift of your female body. Expand your connection to this place within and witness the power, spirit, and joy that energize your life.

....

A MODERN-DAY DILEMMA: PROLONGED SITTING AND PELVIC STAGNATION

Working with women's bodies, I see how our increasingly sedentary lives affect pelvic stagnation and congestion. Literally, the pressure of sitting reduces the blood and cellular flow to the pelvic muscles and organs. This stagnation means that our pelvic muscles may be less robust going into the birth process. Additionally, our routine focus away from our bodies and creative cycles adds to the stagnancy of our creative centers.

Ideally, a woman preparing for pregnancy would first receive internal pelvic massage to increase the health and dynamic potential of the pelvic muscles and bring her attention back to her center. However, whenever a woman restores physical and energetic alignment to the core, her pelvic health becomes more robust.

....

Addressing Specific Effects from Birthing

Birth is a powerful event. The process of moving a baby through your pelvis can have a wide variety of effects on your pelvic balance and function—at least until you receive internal pelvic massage to address these effects. Whether you have a fast birth that challenges your body with the rapid pace or a slow birth where the prolonged pressure or force of pushing impacts the vagina and pelvis, you may experience changes that feel unsettling. Again, even having a cesarean birth can affect pelvic alignment due to the stresses placed on the uterus and other organs during the surgery.

One of my clients said that birth altered her "vaginal confidence." In the next section, I explain the specific effects of birth and describe the gentle treatments that can help restore full vaginal confidence in every woman who gives birth. Though this section focuses on the physical effects of birth, the realignment of the pelvic bowl benefits from both physical and energy processes of bodywork. The pelvic bowl has a physical structure, but any imbalance in the physical space affects the energy flow; likewise, aligning the energy supports physical wellness and vitality.

Anterior Vaginal Stretch

During birth, the baby passes downward through the pelvic bowl and vaginal canal. As this movement occurs, the vagina's anterior wall, posterior wall, or both can be stretched. The pelvic muscles also stretch to accommodate the baby's passage. Many of these "stretch effects" lessen with time. However, they can also persist. A stretch in the front of the vaginal wall can cause the bladder to prolapse or move into this anterior space. Technically this bladder prolapse is called a cystocele.

A change in bladder position that occurs with a cystocele can create a range of symptoms: urinary urgency (needing to go to the bathroom right away), urine leakage, difficulty emptying the bladder, recurrent bladder infections, dribbling urine after urination, and the sense of vaginal pressure or of something pressing out of your vagina. When women find a cystocele for themselves, it can be upsetting, particularly because there is little education for women regarding the physical effects and processes of birth.

A cystocele is relatively common postpartum, but if you search this term on the internet, you will typically only find information about how to correct it surgically. In my healthcare practice, I have helped many women recover from a cystocele by using gentle pelvic-floor bodywork or vaginal massage to rebalance the internal pelvis. Though a slight anterior cystocele may still be palpable, vaginal massage improves overall bladder position. Initially, rest is the best medicine to heal and prevent all types of prolapse. Then bodywork assists the body's natural healing, which includes cellularly repairing the internal bruising or swelling that often occurs from the birth process.

At about six to eight weeks postpartum, I recommend finding a women's health physical therapist or Holistic Pelvic Care practitioner to receive vaginal massage, or more technically termed, myofascial release. With a cystocele, not only is the anterior wall of the vagina stretched, but the fascia or sheath layer of connective tissue that supports the vaginal walls and organ alignment is often out of balance. The fascial layer typically does not adjust on its own, but vaginal work addresses the fascial imbalances and reduces or eliminates the cystocele and resulting bladder symptoms. Working with the fascia reduces the anterior stretch on the vagina and promotes a return to optimal pelvic alignment.

On an energetic level, tension and imbalance in the anterior pelvis can be related to unresolved fears. Acknowledging fear and bringing breath to the anterior pelvis can support the release of these held energies and resulting tension patterns.

Posterior Vaginal Stretch

The posterior wall of the vagina can be stretched as well. In this case, the rectum falls into this new space and makes a rectocele. If you experience difficulty having a bowel movement and find that you have to push to relieve yourself as if constipated, a rectocele is the likely cause. Likewise, with the combination of a rectocele and stretched pelvic muscles, you can have some bowel leakage.

If you are having difficulty with your bowel movements, the first thing to do is refrain from pushing to relieve your bowels, as this increases the rectocele. Instead, place your thumb into the vagina during a bowel movement. Place light pressure on the posterior wall of the vagina to help support the rectum. Inside, you will feel a bulge from the stool pressing into the stretched vaginal wall.

By supporting the bulge with your internal pressure, you actually help the stool move into the central rectum and assist the body in healing and restoring normal alignment. Instead of adding to the stretch by pushing your bowels, you are resetting the fibers into the proper position by giving them support to prevent the over-stretched position on the posterior vaginal wall. As with all pelvic symptoms, rest as much as possible and see a practitioner (after at least six weeks postpartum) to address the fascial imbalances.

Energetically, imbalances in the posterior pelvic bowl can be related to a lack of support. Among high-functioning modern women, there is a tendency to block the support available because receiving it seems to be a sign of weakness. By reaccessing our feminine ability to receive, we gain the capacity to accept the support we crave and deserve.

Pelvic Prolapse

The term *prolapse* simply means that the pelvic organs are moving toward the base of the pelvic bowl or vaginal opening. Prolapse can refer to the bladder, the rectum, or the uterus. I have found that bladder and rectal prolapses are most common after giving birth because the anterior or posterior wall (and fascia) of the vagina become stretched. A uterine prolapse is more rare, occurring when the ligaments become stretched.

If a woman engages in vigorous exercise or jumps on a trampoline in the months following birth, she can cause a uterine prolapse. Due to the central position of the uterus in the pelvic bowl, uterine prolapses are more challenging to reverse. Typically it requires pelvic work as well as Maya Abdominal Therapy, a technique pioneered by Rosita Arvigo to restore the alignment of the uterus. You can find additional information on the internet about the Arvigo techniques of Maya Abdominal Therapy and locate practitioners. More commonly, when a woman feels something prolapsing into her vaginal canal after birth, it is the bladder. Any symptoms of prolapse are a call from the body to rest more and rebuild energy reserves.

Imbalanced Pelvic Muscles and Vaginal Gas

Another common postpartum complaint is a sense of vaginal gas or air passing into and then out of the vagina. Women often discover this symptom several months postpartum, when they return to yoga and attempt some of the inversion poses. As they come out of the pose, the sound of air escaping from the vagina can be a source of embarrassment. This is a sign that pelvic imbalance is inhibiting proper closure of the muscles.

In a healthy pelvic flow, the muscles work dynamically throughout the day and with all the various positions we assume. The coordinated engagement, or synergy, of the pelvic muscles prevents air from entering the vagina. Some of the inversion poses in yoga challenge and strengthen the pelvic floor. When pelvic muscles are imbalanced from the stretch effects of birthing, they are unable to fully engage, and the result is vaginal gas or the inability to control gas from the bowels.

A lack of pelvic muscle synergy does not typically resolve on its own. It is not simply a strengthening of the pelvic muscles that is required, but rather a core rebalancing, including energetic support to integrate the profound physical and energetic transformation. Kegels are a helpful strengthening exercise, but, again, most pelvic problems are not simply a result of pelvic muscle weakness but of core imbalance. Kegels will not resolve a core muscle imbalance. Vaginal massage by a skilled practitioner restores pelvic balance; then Kegels can be used as a part of a strengthening routine. I have assisted many yoga practitioners, whose symptoms of vaginal gas typically resolve with one or two sessions of vaginal massage and core energy rebalancing, to restore their dynamic center—and their yogic peace of mind.

Episotomy and Vaginal Tearing

In the recent past, an episiotomy was performed "preventatively" as a controlled cut while birthing to avoid vaginal tearing. However, women were found to heal more easily with a tear rather than a cut. The edges of torn tissue knit together more readily than those of a straight-line cut. In the case of significant tearing, a stitch repair is necessary and surgeons are well trained to make an in-depth pelvic repair. The new vaginal tissue that arises from a healed tear or stitches can be less flexible than it was originally, causing possible irritation or pelvic pain, but well-done repairs are beneficial.

A woman may worry that she will never be the same. However, internal massage restores pliability and sensation to the place of vaginal healing. In working with thousands of women, I have found the pelvic fascia and vagina have robust healing potential— the female body is well designed for having babies. Receiving pelvic massage stimulates the body's natural healing potential, returning the dynamic quality to vaginal tissue and the core pelvis.

Cesarean Births and Pelvic Symptoms

When a woman has a cesarean birth, she may be surprised by the effects on her vagina and pelvic floor, since she did not have a baby pass fully through her vaginal canal. Sadly, I have even seen misinformation promoting cesareans as a way to preserve the health of the pelvic floor. Though sometimes necessary and potentially life-saving, cesarean birth entails all the risk of surgery as well as potentially profound impacts on the pelvic floor.

Cesarean birth places significant stress on the uterus, uterine ligaments, and core fascia—all of which have connections into the pelvic floor and vagina. The process of lifting the baby from the uterus or pulling on the uterus itself often strains the core pelvis. Or, if the cesarean happens after attempting birth vaginally, there is a force on the fascia from pulling the baby back out of the vaginal canal. The cesarean incision can cause scarring and create a cut in the chi lines of the body; both can be addressed with gentle massage and acupuncture at the incision site.

Recovery from a cesarean is affected by a woman's fatigue level going into the surgery, her body's response to the surgery, and her own feelings about having a cesarean. A woman can be at peace with the need for a cesarean, but she can also feel let down by her body or even grieve the loss of her experience of a vaginal birth. Birth, like life, is a journey with many unknowns. Though we like to think that if we prepare properly we will have the birth experience we desire, women have shown me that it is more likely that we have to meet and make peace with the experience we encounter. One reason a woman may feel incomplete after a cesarean is that it can interrupt the birth flow between a mother and her child. (See the section on restoring birth energy flow [page 116] to address this energetic imbalance.)

How have pregnancy and birth changed your body or being and affected your creative flow?
Where would you like more healing and support?
How has your sense of self been expanded or transformed?

Vaginal Massage and Pelvic Wellness

Vaginal massage is essential for pelvic wellness. It clears stagnation, increases the vitality of the pelvic organs and muscles, and enhances energy flow. Vaginal massage is particularly essential postpartum because it can restore full internal alignment, alleviating the stretch effects of birth as well as greatly assisting the natural healing potential of the body.

Vaginal massage works primarily by restoring the balance and tensile qualities of the fascia, a thin sheath that covers and provides support to the pelvic organs and muscles. When stretched, the fascia can lose some of the tension that provides support to the core pelvis. The internal fascia of the pelvis can also become adhered, limiting the core muscle balance and blood flow. In my classes, I demonstrate the qualities of fascia by using a piece of Saran Wrap to show how it can be stretched or adhered depending on the directions of force from birthing. Using vaginal massage, a practitioner smoothes and rebalances the fascia as well as the underlying pelvic muscles. This core massage also restores the alignment of the fascia around the bladder and rectum, returning these organs to proper position.

In addition to restoring alignment, vaginal massage clears congestion in the pelvis. Clearing this congestion allows for an increase in cellular flow, assisting tissue repair and vitality. After the prolonged period of pregnancy and the intensity of birthing, the pelvis has tremendous work to do in clearing, repairing, and realigning the pelvic and vaginal tissues, and vaginal massage assists this process.

In my practice of postpartum pelvic care, I have found that vaginal massage resolves most pelvic issues arising from birth. Though many women are told that these pelvic changes are permanent or can only be addressed with surgery, I have witnessed—in countless women and in my own body—that we do not need to live with these pelvic imbalances. By attending to the physical core of their body, many women feel a greater connection to the creative life force in their center. My hope is that physical and energetic medicine becomes a routine part of women's wellness, and that all women feel vital and whole in the root of their female body.

For information about finding a pelvic care practitioner see page 286.

....

POSTPARTUM PELVIC SYMPTOMS THAT RESOLVE
WITH VAGINAL MASSAGE

- Feeling of pelvic heaviness or congestion
- Difficulty engaging pelvic muscles

- Urine leakage or urgency
- Bowel dysfunction
- Vaginal gas (air passing easily into the vagina)
- Pelvic or vaginal pain
- Diminished libido
- Pain with intercourse
- Vaginal dryness or open sensation
- Cystocele (bladder prolapsing into anterior vaginal stretch)
- Urethrocele (urethra prolapsing into anterior vaginal stretch)
- Rectocele (rectum prolapsing into posterior vaginal stretch)

....

Women's Stories:
Healing Postpartum Effects and Restoring Pleasure

Jane came for pelvic care one year after her baby's vaginal birth. She had a series of general postpartum pelvic complaints, including difficulty engaging her pelvic muscles, mild urine leakage with a full bladder, and diminished sexual pleasure. These are all signs of core pelvic imbalance that can arise after birthing a baby.

Assessing Jane's pelvis, I could see that her pelvic muscles had an imbalanced engagement pattern. The pelvic muscles on the right side were overcompensating for a decreased engagement on the left. With this imbalanced pattern, the pelvic muscles were not engaging in a coordinated manner. A core imbalance often leaves a woman feeling drained because her root is not providing ample physical and energetic support. Though Jane had no direct complaints of pelvic pain, she also had multiple tender areas (trigger points) in the pelvic muscles that also suggested a pattern of imbalance.

Beginning the vaginal massage, I found that Jane's pelvic fascia began to release and unwind. Jane breathed more deeply and shared that she realized how much she had been "holding it together" in caring for her baby and learning a new routine as a mother. Some excess heat on the right side of her pelvis began to release as well. Excess heat on the right pelvis, near the right ovary, corresponds to a pattern of excess doing. Releasing this energy would help Jane come back to a balanced center, which would benefit both her body and her mothering.

I reminded Jane that her mothering workload would last decades and that she needed to pace herself by building in daily periods of rest and seeking pleasure as a form of renewal. Forging ahead each day was a recipe for burnout and would deplete the sustenance of her own body. Likewise, exhausting herself left little desire for connecting with her partner or having sex. Sex is a wonderful core massage, but it requires sufficient energy.

I continued to work with Jane's core fascial and pelvic balance until the trigger points were significantly reduced and the vital energy had returned. After the massage, she was able to do a Kegel and engage her muscles in a full and coordinated motion. Muscles that move in a coordinated manner will continue to strengthen and reduce pelvic symptoms, engaging naturally and supporting posture throughout the day. At the close of the session, Jane felt a renewed vitality in her own core and more hope for accessing her sense of pleasure.

Postpartum Sex, Libido, and Connection

The year after birthing a baby, the hormones that increase your milk supply also serve to dampen your libido. This is Mother Nature's birth control, reducing the potential of another pregnancy while you are still recovering from childbirth and breastfeeding your baby.

In the postpartum year, it is common to have less interest in lovemaking, decreased vaginal lubrication, and more challenge in having an orgasm; however, there should be some ability and desire to experience pleasure with your partner. If your desire and sense of pleasure is completely flat, it is likely that pelvic imbalances are playing a role and diminishing the blood, energy, and hormonal flow in the pelvis. A woman's pleasure can also be decreased by any irritation in the pelvic fascia, imbalances in the pelvic muscles, and less pliable scar tissue at the vaginal opening—all of which can be addressed with vaginal massage.

Pelvic Imbalances and the Effects on Sex

A robust libido and ability to achieve orgasm require adequate flow in the core and mobility in the pelvic and vaginal tissues. Pregnancy may bring a heightened libido or ability to orgasm because of the increased pelvic flow. Alternately, the imbalances that occur in the pelvic muscles and fascia after vaginal and cesarean birth can reduce hormone and blood flow, cause congestion that dampens sensation, and restrict mobility of the tissues. This wreaks havoc on a woman's sex life. When a woman comes to see me nine months or a year (or longer) postpartum and reports hardly having sex, I know we have work to do for her own well-being and her partnership.

Sex can be a wonderful massage for the pelvic muscles, clearing congestion and increasing blood flow. Orgasm brings blood and the vital flow of chi right to the core of the female body. However, if there is congestion already blocking her libido, a woman will often avoid sex, further increasing the stagnation in her pelvic bowl. Not only does this affect her sex life, but it also means that her pelvic health is compromised. A lack of sex decreases the energy flow in the body and the energy flowing between intimate partners.

How has your sex life changed after having a baby?

What issues do you need more support with?

How can you increase the frequency of your sex and other access to pleasure?

Postpartum Pelvic Pain with Sex

After birthing, women can also experience pain at the vaginal opening. This pain signals a fascial imbalance or restriction in the scar tissue formed from any tearing or stitches. It makes sex quite painful. Trying to push through this pain by having sex anyway is awkward and often increases tension in the pelvic muscles. Alternately, avoiding sex will not alleviate the problem. Restrictions in the pelvic fascia impede blood and energy flow to the core, causing vaginal pain or tightness in the tissues. This pent-up pelvic congestion will reduce overall pelvic vitality until addressed by skilled vaginal massage techniques. After the massage, women often realize how much tension had accumulated and are relieved to feel a more normal sense of circulation in the vagina and pelvis.

Without skilled care, some women just learn to live with the pain, even avoiding sex altogether. The issue is not simply a lack of sex, though; the tension pattern in the pelvic floor limits the overall health of the muscles, skin, and pelvic organs. For a woman's long-term pelvic health, it is essential to address this pain and tension pattern.

Imagine a knot of tension in the shoulders, and then imagine this in the core of your pelvis. This internal place sets the tone in the center of your being; if you feel dynamic, then your energy arises from this place. Core health is essential for your vibrance, creative flow, and centered wellness—all of which are vital for mothering. If you have symptoms of pelvic pain or discomfort postpartum, seek out a women's health practitioner. A practitioner can address the fascial imbalances, pelvic imbalances, perineal irritation from stitches or scarring, and pelvic tension points that may be contributing to the pain. If you have any prolonged and deeper pelvic pain involving touch to the uterus or unexpected bleeding beyond the initial six weeks, have your provider check for a uterine infection. Postpartum pain should be resolved and pleasure restored.

Exercise: Restoring Your Sacred Sensuality

The changes in the vagina, belly, breasts, or overall body may cause a woman to feel self-conscious or even ashamed. Feeling unattractive is a serious libido dampener. Working with a pelvic care practitioner can lessen some of the pelvic changes and restore a sense of vitality in the core. Be gentle with your body. Attend to yourself. Find clothing that fits well, in colors that appeal to your palette, even as your body rebalances. Do what makes you feel good. Remember that you have created a life; attend to yourself as a sacred goddess.

1. Close your eyes and notice the sensations in your body. Where do you feel strong and radiant? Where is your body in need of tending?

2. Ask your body what it craves, and make space for these bodily desires in your daily life.

3. Spend the next five minutes paying attention to your senses. Notice where you feel alert and where you need to awaken your sensory system. What do you see? What do you hear? How do you feel? Pay attention to your skin sensations as well as your deeper senses. Move your body and notice how the movement feels.

4. Bless your body: *May I restore my radiant form. May I be well and fully nourished. May my whole body be blessed. May I know the sacredness of my body.*

5. After these blessings, notice how your body responds. Remember your sacred body. Awaken to the sensual nature that invites pleasure into your days.

A Changing Partnership: Honoring Your Differences

Carrying a baby and traveling to the spirit door is life altering for you and your intimate relationship with your partner. Nothing brings lineage issues to the surface like becoming parents. The stress and tension of parenting, combined with the lineage of mothering or fathering each of you has received, makes all your issues more visible. It is imperative to nurture not only your own well-being but also the well-being of your partnership.

In addition to the other life changes, postpartum hormones can intensify both the feelings of connection and conflict. In my practice, a common complaint I hear from women is that they find themselves feeling angry with their partner, sometimes without even knowing the reason. Keep some perspective while the feelings roll through. Monitor your reactions and remember that your feelings may be greater than the truth of what is happening in the moment. Also, you and your partner have been through a tremendous change, which requires time to adjust. Being patient and ultra-loving with one another is a high priority. In order to strengthen your bond even while in the midst of this transition, focus on your partner's attributes and the traits that attract you. Enjoy your baby together, and savor the union that will nurture this new life.

Some of the early conflicts that arise between mothers and fathers are gender differences in caretaking. Of course, individual parents will vary in many ways, even among mothers or fathers, but the gender issues arise often enough to be worth mentioning. A perfect example of this comes from my own experience. When my first son was six months old, I took him to an infant massage class to learn techniques for baby massage. Most of the participants were mothers. On the last day, partners—most of whom were fathers—were invited to attend.

My husband's ranching family is less comfortable hugging or touching one another, and perhaps being male accentuated my husband's discomfort with touch. Still, I wanted him to be different with his own children. During the instruction of the massage technique, my husband's hand had only partial contact with our son's body. He seemed to be doing the massage halfheartedly. By the end of the class, I was fuming. I felt that my husband was already well on his way to passing down a lack of touch and all the issues that came with it. Though we can pass on patterns of wounding while parenting our children, in this case, I had loaded meaning onto one situation.

I approached the instructor after class and shared some of my concerns, asking if she might talk to my husband about the importance of touch. Instead of speaking to my partner, she told me an ancient story about how mothers hold their children close and teach them about themselves, while fathers hold their children up to the sky and teach them about their relationship to the world. This was not what I wanted to hear. Though I pondered her words, I did not truly comprehend the meaning until a few more years of parenting had passed and I gained an appreciation for the attributes of different parenting styles.

As a mother, I was innately attuned to my children's needs, so much in fact that I often intuited a need just as they were beginning to ask for something. To have a need met by their father, these same children had to become much louder or even ask for something multiple times to receive his attention. In a way, he was less sensitive to their needs, which meant that they had to learn the essential skill of advocating for themselves. Our skills as parents complemented each other. In the presence of too little sensitivity, a child can become overly frustrated in trying to communicate. However, with only sensitive parenting, they do not learn to be self-aware or to self-advocate because their needs are met so readily. Though mothers and fathers can switch these types of roles, typically mothers are the more sensitive ones and the most intimate caretakers of a child.

In same-sex partners, gender differences may not play as strong a role, but parenting styles can still differ. A couple can increase their communication and skill set by respecting the benefits of their different styles. Ideally, couples learn from each other, and their collective strengths offset the inevitable places of lack. It is worth talking about concerns and identifying the limiting patterns, just as I continued to advocate for the importance of touch and connection in our home. But both parents do not need to provide the same things for their children.

Differing parenting styles can expand, rather than restrict, the learning for a child who will need to get along with many types of people. One parent can also choose alternate styles to be responsive for a range of needs. A more feminine style of parenting is nurturing and intuitive, while a masculine style is more playful and rowdy. Both genders can access their feminine or masculine aspects for a specific situation or their child's present needs. Remember that you and your partner are a parenting team, and that flexibility with one another and your children increases your parenting capacity.

What are the strengths or challenges of your parenting skills?
How do these strengths and challenges coincide with or complement those of your partner?
How can you honor one another and work together effectively?

Reviving Your Access to Pleasure

Beyond parenting, remember that your partnership is built upon a connection with one another. Though parenting can easily become your primary focus, find your way back to your connection as partners. The transition to parenting and the added stress can leave you feeling unsure of how to be in relationship. Just as it takes time to learn how to be parents, it takes time to redefine your way of being together. Rather than focusing on points of stress or what is lacking, identify and communicate your needs. Take efforts to restore your union; make it a priority to find pleasure with your partner.

One of the best cures for a libido or partner connection that has gone dormant is to seek daily sources of pleasure. You can reawaken your sensual nature by taking baths, wearing a plush robe, eating with pleasure in mind, and generally savoring the senses. Try something new with your partner, such as a date or concert in an unexplored venue. Expand your sexual play with some inspired reading or a field trip to your local female-friendly sex shop. Explore your G-spot and find more ways to access pleasure. In my practice, I have noticed that women who make sexual pleasure a priority seem happier and more relaxed.

When sex is pleasurable, it revitalizes and relieves tension in your pelvic muscles—it is the ultimate pelvic massage. Orgasms increase blood, hormonal, and cellular flow in the whole body. If you are not having orgasms, skilled vaginal massage by a pelvic care practitioner can restore the alignment and flow that supports your sexual pleasure. One of my clients felt "broken" after having her second baby; she found that sex hurt and orgasms were elusive. In one session of pelvic care, we restored the energetic and physical alignment in her core pelvis. She stood up and remarked how much better she felt. I suggested she might want to take a "test drive." A few days later, I received a message saying that she had "taken her new car out and had four orgasms." When I first read her message I thought, *That must be some car*. Then I remembered our session and realized what she was referring to.

You have expanded your body and spirit by becoming a mother. Give yourself permission to expand and explore new things in other aspects of life. Birthing a child is a transformative process that offers new potentials, patterns of embodiment, and ways of being in your relationship. When your world shifts, let it bring in fresh experiences and qualities that enhance your enjoyment of life with those you love. You deserve to feel sexy, mama.

SEVEN

Everyday Mothering from the Center

Mothering is my daily walk in the mystery of life. In the tending of children and home, I bear witness to the sacred in both the simple and significant events we encounter together. When my husband and I were deciding whether to bring a third child into our family, talking about it did not bring about resolution. To become clear for myself, I chose a Maya Abdominal Massage self-care retreat for women to open the necessary ritual space to commune with spirit.

It was a warm summer day in the Oregon countryside when nine of us made a spiritual bath as part of the retreat. This ritual of making a spiritual bath has since become a part of our family repertoire of energy medicine (see page 13). At the retreat, our group of women spread themselves apart on the dry field behind the farmhouse, each one with her own thoughts and wildflower-infused bowl of water. I placed my towel on the ground, and settled into the peace of the quiet air and the caress of the sun on my bare skin. I began to splash the air around me, and a bee joined my movements. Then another bee came, and another.

At first I was frightened, having learned to resist the sensation of a bee against the skin. But then I noticed that the bees were gently bumping me. I followed their movements while splashing the spirit water. I found myself swaying from side to side. I was moving in a figure-eight motion, lifting one arm up and around and then shifting to the other side and lifting the other arm up and around. Repeating a cyclical motion from side to side, we became one, a growing field of twenty or thirty bees and I, swaying rhythmically together.

The spiritual bath clears and aligns the energy field. With the bath of wildflowers and the bees, my field of energy became crystalized air around me. Lifting my towel to dry my skin, I saw the bees fly one by one into a hole that my towel had been covering.

The women and I moved inside for the second aspect of our ritual, listening to a guided womb meditation by Rosita Arvigo. As mentioned previously, Arvigo is a master herbalist, traditional healer, and the founder of the Arvigo Techniques of Maya Abdominal Therapy, a wellness practice that helps women and men restore health and balance in the pelvis and core body. In the Maya tradition, physical, herbal, and spiritual medicine are combined—and with profound effects. I lay down in my bright energy field to listen to Arvigo's voice.

I have little memory of the words said, only that I had two clear visions. In the first, I was giving birth in the "fire room" ritual space of our basement, joined by my husband and two sons. In the second, I was walking into a class with Rosita Arvigo while carrying a baby. The visions were strong and immediate; I knew I had received my answer regarding a third child.

From my experience, visions can be inspiring but can also serve as a call to action. The feminine aspect of our nature receives the vision. The masculine aspect works to manifest the vision. Therefore, I left the retreat and called the Arvigo office the next day. Though Arvigo lives in Belize, there is an office based in the United States to coordinate her trainings. I asked if they would like to come to Oregon. My timing was divine; they were looking for a West Coast venue.

The following June, I gave birth in the fire room of our house, with my husband and sons there. In September, I walked into a professional training class with Rosita Arvigo, carrying my third child, a three-month-old son, in my arms.

The realization of these visions is profound, perhaps all the more because we have largely forgotten our ability to visualize and then manifest our visions. We often believe that our creative abilities lie in the hands of others rather than harnessing our creative potential for ourselves and our families.

Savoring Laughter and the Mystery Unfolding

A few months after the Arvigo class, while I was still basking in the glow of mystery unfolding, my oldest son was preparing to receive his first communion. He was seven and had the assignment to create a family crest, making symbols for each of his family members. I watched over his shoulder, seeing the salmon and tree that he made to represent his dad, who works in environmental conservation on salmon issues. I eagerly looked to see what he was making for me. As the lines took shape, I asked him, "What is that, honey?" He said, "It's a bed, Mom, and that's you sleeping." There was indeed a bed and a little round head—me, presumably. He drew large Z's over my head to illustrate me sleeping. Then he drew some symbols for his brothers and announced, "I'm done."

I paused at the image of me asleep in the bed. "Is that all, honey? Are you sure you are done?"

"Yep, I'm done," he assured me.

I guess I needed to be more direct, "A picture of me in bed . . . is that all you can think of for Mama? Is there anything else?"

I knew I sounded desperate. His perspective of me asleep was in utter contrast to the images flashing through my mind—of birthing, nursing, carrying, feeding, playing with him day by day and year upon year. All the bodywork, rituals, outings, and classes that we had done together in the past seven years, and this was how he saw me? Sleeping?

He shrugged and thought hard. "That's all I can think of. You like to sleep in, Mom."

Yes, I thought, I sleep in because I have done night duty for seven years. My husband and I divide every aspect of home and childcare, but night duties fall to me because I can function with disrupted sleep. And I cherish the intimate night hours with my children.

I sighed. "What about drumming?" I asked, thinking of all the times we had traveled to the beach and the boys played on the sand while I played my elk-skin drum. They were sacred times to me, but clearly I would have a different perspective of my mothering than my children would.

The magnitude of this was sinking in. My son exclaimed, "Yeah, drumming! I'll draw a drum for you."

I laughed. Who says you can't at least influence a child's perspective? He finished a salmon and tree for his dad, a rocket ship for one brother, a blanket for his baby brother, and a drum and a bed with "zzzz" for me. Though it seemed a little like cheating, I laughed hard enough to shed tears when I shared the story with my fellow mothers in my book club. In the face of our myths and expectations for mothering, at times all you can do is laugh.

The reality is we are in service to our children. All our hard and joyous work in tending them may go unrecognized because what we do is woven into the fabric of their lives. Of course we can encourage attributes of gratitude, but to appreciate our mothering, they will have to go far enough away from us to gain perspective—someday long into the future. We ourselves must remember that the day-to-day tending is slowly making a bountiful life.

The task of mothering children reminds me of *The Painted Drum* by Louise Erdrich. In the story, there is a man whose entire life is spent tending a grove of trees that will be made into a sacred drum when he is no longer alive. In mothering, we are tending the seeds of the sacred. Because we may scarcely witness the results of our tending, our satisfaction must arise from the sacred act of our tending. This is easier said than done, as I discovered in responding to my son's family-crest project.

That night, while my younger sons were asleep next to me and my husband was downstairs reading the newspaper, my oldest son climbed into my bed to talk and have some rare one-on-one mama time. Tucked under the warm covers, our faces close together, I thought that perhaps a bed—with a mother included—was the perfect symbol for all that mothering entails.

Resources for Whole-Child Care

Taking care of a child is like weaving a great tapestry; it starts with a simple thread and, through day-to-day tending over a long period of time, evolves into an intricate creation. In the process of weaving a life with your child, you will develop many resources by mothering from the wisdom of your own center. Every woman's female center contains a wealth of creative resources. Though there is a plethora of books and other information to read about parenting, in applying the information, I always point a woman back to her own center: *What does your intuition say?* You contain the energy for your child; your center has wisdom for this unique soul and how they are to be cared for.

Making a routine from your child's many unpredictable needs, which vary each day, is a puzzle. Instead of a specific schedule, create an organic rhythm that alternates between active and quiet periods. Take a walk in the fresh air and then come inside for quiet reading, nursing, or a nap. Follow a flow pattern that moves out and then in again, responding to the energy of your mothering day. For any mother who has been in the working world, where continuous production is emphasized, finding a more natural rhythm is a fundamental shift, but it is one that will serve for a lifetime. We were meant to move in organic and seasonal rhythms.

In developing your rhythm, include time to connect with others. Set up a light schedule for you and your child that incorporates community activities like a music class, reading time at the library, or a mothering group. The early days of mothering can be isolating, so it is essential to have a few scheduled activities where you can interface with other mothers.

Find a Quality Naturopath and Cranial-Sacral Practitioner

I learned how to tend a child with a fever or other illness and how to support their immune system from holistic practitioners of naturopathy. At first I responded to my children's illnesses with fear and worry. With the guidance of a skilled practitioner, I came to cherish these "downtimes" of caring for my child with holistic immune support, recognizing that the illness was actually helping to build their immunity. A naturopath can also assist you in navigating serious illness or even the vaccination debate. The website GenerationRescue.org has helpful information from some thoughtful medical providers about alternative vaccine schedules as well.

Cranial-sacral bodywork is an osteopathic practice of care designed to align the body. It is gentle and effective for babies and young children. Many different types of providers may practice cranial-sacral bodywork; look for a practitioner who specializes in working with children. Because I'm a proponent of physical medicine, my children have received routine bodywork for wellness, as well as in response to any significant fall or injury. They know the power of physical medicine in healing their own bodies. Just as with women's health, physical medicine is both a missing ingredient and powerful tool for pediatric wellness. Cranial-sacral therapy was essential medicine after my infant son's serious fall (and resulting cranial fracture), and it helped a friend's child recover more fully from a brain injury. Another type of osteopathic bodywork is visceral manipulation. This can be helpful in addressing the health of the viscera or abdominal organs. If your child has any type of abdominal surgery, find a practitioner skilled in visceral manipulation through the Barral Institute.

Another bodywork technique that I recommend is Qigong Sensory Massage. Pioneered by Dr. Louisa Silva, who has dual degrees as a medical doctor and Chinese medicine practitioner, this is a parent-based massage technique done along the meridians (or energy lines) of a child's body. It supports the immune system and development and addresses issues of autism and sensory integration (the ability to process sensory information). When children have frequent tantrums and other difficulties processing stimuli or making transitions, this type of bodywork is tremendously helpful for increasing a child's physical and energetic capacity. Rather than seeing these issues as purely behavioral, parents can draw upon this type of massage to ease a child's bodily discomfort or energy blocks and effectively increase overall resiliency (and thus behavior). The technique can be learned by DVD and booklet, and there is a growing network of practitioners trained to support parents and address specific health concerns. (Find out more at qsti.org.)

I found Dr. Silva while searching for healthcare for my second son, who was exposed over several winters, along with the rest of our family, to a gas leak in our furnace. Though our family became sick, we recovered primarily with the assistance of holistic medicine. However, some of the toxic effects persisted for my second son, as he was an infant during the exposure period. The Qigong Sensory Massage helped clear the toxins from his body and vastly improved his energy, sensory regulation, and overall health. Dr. Silva also shares from her Chinese medicine perspective that because of the energy flow between parents and children, parents have an innate healing ability in regard to using touch with their children. My husband and I have incorporated the massage for each of our children to increase core vitality, and they frequently request it as part of their bedtime routine.

Expand Your Parenting Skills

While there are many parenting books that can add to your skill set, there are some essential titles that fundamentally shifted my own parenting. For the first year, I recommend Aletha Solter's book *The Aware Baby*, in which she provides a holistic perspective for addressing your child's basic needs: crying/expression, sleep/ rest, food/nourishment, play/learning, respect, and attachment. Perhaps most important, Solter also details the ways that parents' own past wounds in these certain areas can affect their ability to meet those basic needs. It is humbling and fascinating to learn how, in certain areas, your challenges with your children mirror your own childhood issues. Working on these issues brings healing.

The Aware Baby is a particularly valuable resource for identifying previously unmet needs in yourself and then providing more fully for your child. I had an "aha" moment while reading Solter's fresh perspective about crying. I had assumed that being a good mother involved quieting and calming my child, soothing his cries so that he stopped crying. Solter offers the perspective that children may need to cry to release stress and emotions. I incorporated these techniques into my parenting so that part of my comfort involved listening to my children's cries while holding them.

Solter suggests that you never stop a child's cry or distract him or her from the tears. However, I found that I could only listen attentively to a crying child if my own needs were met. If I was tired or hungry, it served us better for me to say, "I know that you are upset right now. I'm going to make dinner so that we can eat. Let's share more feelings later." A balanced approach allowed me to listen to my children but also attend to my own needs or the needs of the family.

Learn about Child Development

Learning about child development, beginning in the toddler years, will ensure that you have the skills to work with your child at each age. One of my essential resources is a series of books titled *Your One-Year-Old, Your Two-Year-Old, Your Three-Year-Old*, and so on, by Louise Bates Ames et al. and the Gesell Institute of Human Development. Written in the early 1980s, the books' language is a bit dated, but the descriptions of behavioral stages of development are thoroughly insightful.

Each of the books has a theme that serves as its subtitle. For instance, the subtitle of *Your Three-Year-Old* is *Friend or Enemy*, because children this age tend to perceive the world with a black-and-white perspective. Though every child enters these age-related stages at their own pace, knowing the themes that arise in each developmental stage makes them less personal and more a regular part of a child's progression.

Understanding childhood development also eases the stress that comes with the changes in your child. For example, when my first son was three-and-a-half years old and started to act as if I were his enemy, saying things like "I hate you," I was initially alarmed. Seeing this in my first son, I thought that something was wrong in my parenting or that we might be heading toward a difficult relationship. A friend suggested the Gesell books, and I read about the "friend or enemy" stance of many children at this age. Reading that his behavior was normal for a child his age allowed me to stay more neutral about it instead of projecting a particular meaning onto the behavior.

By the time my third son was entering the "friend or enemy" stage, I had no personal reaction at all. I knew it was a normal developmental stage and that it would pass. I had the confidence of a parent who has been through several stages with other children and developed skills to engage them. He might say to me, "I hate you," or "I'm never ever going to like you," and I would take him in my arms, saying, "Is it hard to hear me say no?" or "Is it hard to be the youngest one in the family?" Or I would even be silly with him: "I'll bet you'd like me to say yes to everything you ask for." Instead of reacting to his words, I communicated with the energy beneath them, identifying the frustration that he was feeling but did not have the words for. In response to being heard in this way, his body would typically soften, and he might say, "Let's read a book, Mama," or "I love you, Mama."

Understand Patterns of Development

The other key point from the Gesell Institute books is that children tend to move through patterns of development, alternating periods of disequilibrium—when things may seem more difficult and turbulent as they prepare to master new skills—and then equilibrium, when they move with more confidence and ease. These periods roughly correlate to a year, with six months of progressive disequilibrium and then six months of progressive equilibrium. By paying attention over time, you will notice the relevance of these patterns. With our multiple children, I find that they are at different places in this continuum, so one may be having more challenges and be in a period of disequilibrium while another is in a period of relative calm and flow.

Rather than labeling children as challenging, it is helpful to recognize patterns of development that occur for all children. If a child is in a difficult stage, he or she often requires more support and patience. As a parent, knowing that this behavior is a stage of development rather than a personality trait can be helpful information. Also, these stages pass. If one child is in an integrative phase, he or she may be able to assist the family and bring more ease so that there is space for the child who is building new skills. Over the course of a year, children will evolve to a new phase of development, so that the first child is now challenged by the skill-building phase while the previously stressed child rests into a sense of skills mastered.

Around age three, children begin to feel and become aware of their powerful feelings. They also begin to separate from the mother-baby energy field and establish their own energetic space. As such, it is helpful to build language regarding emotions so that children can understand their emotions in a positive manner—as strong energy that moves through and serves to guide us. Two of my favorite books for young children are *Today I Feel Silly and Other Moods That Make My Day*, by Jamie Lee Curtis, and *Glad Monster, Sad Monster*, by Ed Emberley and Anne Miranda. Both of these books explore feelings in a playful and thoughtful manner. Reading books with children can be a safe way for them to understand emotions and other aspects of themselves, witness social interactions, and have a basic emotional framework to bring to their ever-expanding world.

As your children develop a healthy capacity for emotional expression, you may also be required to take on personal work regarding any wounds you have in your own emotional realm. This is tender and vulnerable ground but worth exploring. To give a wider range of expression for your children, you must be comfortable with full expression for yourself.

Create Your Tribe

Mothering was never meant to be a solo endeavor. Though many mothers live within the context of the nuclear family, it is wise to create a tribe. A tribe can include friends and other mothers, extended family, neighbors, babysitters, wellness practitioners, teachers, and even animal companions in your home. In a tribe, each member has a role, so the work is shared. Creating your own tribe of support is essential for providing for your children without trying to be everything yourself. As your children grow, they also take their place in giving service to the tribe and community based on their gifts. A mother can mobilize and coordinate the connections and the caretaking by drawing upon the collective resources of the tribe.

Among mothers, as in any group, skills vary by individual. Together, we can offer more by accessing the natural potential of a particular mother. In my own community, I have learned from mothers who excel at play, teaching, making food or natural remedies, and utilizing organizational skills. At the same time, I share my own tools of energy medicine and family ritual. In a tribe, every member is valued for his or her unique contribution. Know your own skills and recognize those of the mothers and others in your midst.

Years ago at a conference, I heard Sobonfu Somé, a ritual leader from the Dagara tribe in Africa, speak about her experience growing up in a tribe. Her perspective was astonishing to my Western mind. Somé was about four years old before she realized that she had come from one woman's body. Imagine being held by a group of women in this profound way. Celebrating the skills of our co-mothers and letting our children be held by them can bridge an unnatural divide and ease the mothering load.

Make It Fun

Having children is an invitation for fun—or it ought to be. As the mother, you maintain and cultivate the family flow and can direct it toward fun. If you enjoy playing games, bring this into your mothering. If you like to go on walks, plan your day around being outside. If you love ritual, incorporate this into your mothering days. Based on what you love, take your children to musical events, art classes, or children's museums—your children will eagerly follow. It does not matter what you are doing; if you are having fun, so will they.

Whether you enjoy animals, road trips, spiritual events, holidays, big parties, intimate dinners, dancing, dressing up, playing soccer, reading Harry Potter books aloud, watching funny movies, baking, eating out, hiking in the woods, or exploring neighborhood coffee shops, move with your children toward whatever fuels your fun, and mothering will be the joy it is intended to be.

Bring your dynamic essence and passion as a creative being to your mothering. Sometimes women have a limited imprint of mothering, restricted by a certain way of being. Yet our children want to be held in the fullness of our bright potential. Just like each child, you are a blessing. The joy arises when you give form to your unique expression in each moment of your mothering journey.

Motherhood as a Centering Practice

My primary recommendation for mothering is to learn how to read and work with the energy of your own body—and then mother from the potential of your own center. Whether you are a stepmother, adoptive mother, birth mother, or co-mother, these essentials for mothering from the center include physical touch, the energy connection with your child, and the blessing energy from spirit. Drawing upon the creative energy of your center for mothering will strengthen your connection and access to this potential within. In this way, motherhood can become a centering practice for aligning oneself with the divine energy that is meant to flow through the body. I work with mothers to access this core creative energy and I draw upon it for all my mothering. With the intense demands of mothering, every mother needs to be able to use the resources from her own creative reservoir.

These centering tools increase the flow of joyful energy in the mother-child relationship and ease the stress. If I find myself in a place of stress with one or more of my children, I use touch, energy medicine, and blessings to readjust our connection. For example, after centering myself, I reach out to physically touch my children. I then place my attention on the energy connection between us (calling to mind the birth energy flow), and with blessings, I invite the assistance of spirit: *May we find our connection. May peace be restored. May love surround us.*

Physical touch is soothing and brings us back into connection with our bodies. Feeling the energy connection between ourselves and our children brings fresh chi, or energy, to our bond with one another, even when we are struggling. Blessings call helpful energies to any situation and assist the alignment of the overall energy field.

If I find that even with my essential mothering tools, our family keeps returning to these stress points, I evaluate the bigger picture. Am I feeling strained myself or that I'm not receiving enough support? Is my energy system out of balance? Is my child experiencing a particular stress or moving through a stage that requires more support? There may be a larger issue that needs attention, and by sensing the discord, I can begin to address it directly.

There are times in every mother-child pair when the connection is frayed. The first priority in these periods is to tend and repair the connection. It may require that you seek extra help, whether through venting to a friend, working with a counselor, brainstorming with your partner, or finding specific support or resources for your child. It may involve decreasing your overall stress load or increasing positive time together. The main objectives are to realize that there is an issue, to work with any strain patterns, and to assist the love and flow between you. Your connection is the medicine.

A mother who is in tune with her child can hear his or her cry and answer it even if she is busy at the moment: *I hear you. You sound frustrated; what do you need? I'm tired, too, after the long night we had. Let's take a walk; the fresh air will help us.* It's so simple, yet a thousand aspects of the future depend on that thread of connection.

How is your mother-child connection presently?
Are there any points of strain that need attention?
How would you like to nurture and strengthen this
      connection?

A Glimpse into the Profound

In the process of mothering from the center, there is an opportunity to glimpse the profound nature of our lives together, not only as parent and child but also as spiritual beings. Being present in the center assists your ability to witness these sacred moments. When my first son was nearly three years old, his face suddenly became worried and he lay down upon the floor. Then he crawled on his belly, looking to me like a soldier in a war zone. I sat on the floor facing him and opened my arms. He did not seem to see me, so I called to him. His head turned to my voice and he moved rapidly on his belly toward me. Once reaching my arms, he climbed into them and collapsed. Through tears he cried out, "I was in a plane. There was fire. I'm so glad I live here now."

His words sent a shiver through my body. It was as if he had reclaimed some part of his energy from another place. Was this imagination or could he be reliving a past life or a lineage memory of war? I would never know, but I held him and rocked back and forth. "You are safe. You made it," I assured him. A few minutes later he climbed out of my arms and returned to his regular play.

Bearing witness to babies and children as they come into their bodies makes one ponder the nature of being and movement of souls. In my mothering, I have discovered a deeper truth that what we see in our children may reflect layers of energy and experience that are beyond the time and space of the typical senses; that in our time together we may be healing or expanding the energy we have carried as part of our greater soul. In my own experience, the more we accept the multidimensional aspect of being in ourselves and our children, the more we will perceive. A profound example of this is *The Horse Boy*, a book and film documentary by Rupert Isaacson. It is an epic story of Isaacson's quest as a father searching for healing for his son, Rowan, which involves horses, travel to Mongolia, and shaman healers working at the spirit door. And we might all have stories like these if we expand our perception and pay attention to the energy current in the center of ourselves and our children.

The Creative Resources in the Center of Our Bodies
We have abundant creative resources within our bodies that can provide guidance, bring energy when we need it, and restore the mother-child connection. When one of my children is having a difficult time, such as a conflict or high-level frustration, I redirect my awareness away from the situation itself and into my own root. Typically I will find that I am in a reaction pattern: my body is tensing and my energy rising away—as if escaping—from my root and earth connection. When this happens, the energy flow becomes blocked, and often the energy around the heart closes in a protective manner.

When in the midst of a challenging mothering moment, instead of reacting to what is happening, I focus on finding my center and feeling my feet on the ground. I breathe deeply into my connection to the earth and bring more flow into my root. I expand the energy around my bowl and my heart by breathing toward, and then sensing the reserves, in my center. While a head-based response perceives only a "right" or "wrong" approach, the creative womb and loving heart offer infinite options and potential. Typically I feel better just by restoring my root flow. From there, I may be able to better comfort my child, deflate a conflict by taking a different approach, or engage the situation in an entirely new manner.

By taking a moment to reestablish a connection to the creative energy in my center, I also receive the divine support and love that I need in those hard moments. Asking for a blessing for myself can also be helpful: *May I give and receive love in this moment. May peace and helpful energies surround us.* To access these creative resources on a daily basis, it is essential to remember the energy medicine in our centers.

Setting Your Core Intentions

To center yourself in your mothering potential rather than its challenges, direct your creative essence through clear intentions for making a creative motherhood. For example, my top three core intentions for my creative energy include being available to tend my children, nourishing my creative practice, and living in a home and manner that support energy flow. On a given day, I set my agenda around these values.

Since tending my children is a high priority, I work a part-time schedule, with the flexibility to be present for my children. Their needs come before my work. I never leave for work until I feel that they are settled, even though I have been late to the office because I am spending a little extra time soothing a child. I hold my children in my center and schedule work around them, making our connection the priority. If I teach or participate in a workshop that requires an extended period of concentrated work over several days or being out of town, I expect to set down my work when I return in order to reconnect with my children, rather than attempt to do more and catch up on the work I missed during the workshop.

Nourishing my creative practice is also a high priority. This means that I write, make ritual, or even engage my kids in creative ways before I take on housework or other tasks. I receive regular bodywork to enhance my creative flow, and I follow my creative energy in regard to the timing of creative projects. If I feel a strong inspiration and flow, I seize the opportunity and work with it. If my energy feels low, I take a break or even organize the house as a way to clarify my creative space.

Living in a dynamic creative flow is like applying feng shui or energy alignment practices in every aspect of life. With this as a core value, I take regular time to clean and clear clutter in my home and workplace. I also make dates for my husband and me and plan activities to enjoy one another as a family to brighten the overall potential of our family energy field. And when we encounter repeated challenges, I work on realigning the overall flow by initially centering myself and then sensing what needs adjustment or attention.

What are your top three creative intentions?
How do these correlate with the overall energy flow?
How might your intentions change as your life and mothering evolve?

Energy Tools for Children and the Home

The creative essence of your female body is the most powerful tool for cultivating balanced energy in your home and with your children. Knowing how to access and align your own energy center is essential for mothering from this place.

Following the Flow

Rather than a set to-do list that demands a specific order, try organizing your mothering days by following the flow from your center. The particulars of organizing a day, week, or longer period can be based on this flow, which evolves fluidly with the energy of the day or your family's changing needs. For myself, I connect with my center to be able to feel this flow, but then I ride the energy current to the task at hand. Whether I am writing, tending the house, running errands, or planning a family trip, I feel this current and the energy openings from my center. That is how I decide when and where to focus my attention.

It takes practice to sense energy flow. You can start with a small thing, like running a particular errand. Sense from within your center and notice whether you feel an opening of ease, like excitement and potential, or whether you feel congestion and hesitation. If you sense an opening, go ahead and run the errand. The traffic, the people you encounter, even finding what you need will often flow more easily. If you sense congestion but proceed anyway, you may run into traffic or difficulties, or even find that the store is out of your item. Try it and see for yourself.

When we encounter a pattern of congestion, it can be ideal to postpone the task, errand, or trip until a sense of flow is restored. Also, it may be time to organize the home or work space, spend time with family members, or work with your own energy system to support greater flow. Stagnancy can build up if certain aspects of the energy field have been neglected or are in need of attention. Sometimes this means setting down your agenda or letting go of your expectations with respect to timing in order to reestablish the flow.

Your family needs and your overall capacity to meet them have an ebb and flow. Energy alternates between periods of expansive creation and restorative retreat. By coordinating your movements with your energy and incorporating energy practices, you can optimize your flow.

> Do you have a practice for connecting to your center?
> How can you access or cultivate more mothering flow?

Exercise: Engaging Your Center and Sensing the Flow

1. Bring awareness to your creative center: your pelvic bowl, where your creative energy flows. Notice the sensations in your core body. Does your center feel energized or congested? If you have any congestion or imbalances, do the Pelvic Bowl Sings exercise (page 248) before proceeding.

2. Notice the phase of your creative energy and whether it is expansive and moving out toward the world or more dormant and internal. See how your energy is moving and think about how you are presently using it; take note of how you are letting the energy support you and where you might need to adjust your present load to match your energy. Ask yourself, What do I need in order to align myself with this current flow?

3. Now sense each family member. Whose energy is aligning with a flow and whose is out of balance? Notice what is supporting the overall flow and what might be needed to restore balance. Ask yourself, What does my child or my partner need for better flow? (You don't need to do everything, but it's good to reflect on it.)

4. Set two to three intentions for facilitating the family flow. Does the family need more structure, added fun, bodywork, or quality time together? Reinforce the flow by emphasizing ease and adding support as necessary. If you have a specific question

about adding an activity, making a family plan, or receiving some support for a particular issue, set it in the center of this flow pattern and observe the response with your inner eye and senses. Does it increase and align the flow or add congestion? What else is needed? This picture will inform your action and help you make requests from each family member.

5. Finish with a blessing. See the radiance of spirit touching you and each member of the family, aligning the energy. Bringing an alignment to the family field supports the overall flow. Let spirit help you. Say a blessing and then carry the energy with you through the day: *May we be blessed with an abundance of ease and joy in our family.*

Addressing Energy Depletion

Even as you practice finding your center and sensing energy, there are times when, due to depletion, you will not find a flow pattern. When this happens, be kind with yourself. Take a break or go to bed early. The strain of raising children—on you and your partner— is real. The reality is that in many families, both parents are working and there is little external support. Tend to your children's basic needs as best you can, and then take time away from the challenge at hand to address your own needs.

When I am feeling depleted, I tell my children that my patience cup or my energy system is getting low. I will also say, "You can help me refill my well." I provide them with examples: finding peace with one another, helping me clean the house, and being thoughtful. In this way, they recognize that I am doing tremendous work and that they can be empowered to assist the return to balance.

Be sure that you yourself are receiving adequate breaks and fun connection time with your partner, exercise, and rest—because you are running a marathon every day just by mothering. When these self-care tools are in place and you are still struggling to find harmony in your center, then you may require additional help. Your own childhood wounds are often revealed by the experience of parenting. To assist the process of establishing new and supportive ways of being, seek a counselor, receive body and energy work, and make connections with other mothers.

Exercise: Energy Practices for Restoring the Flow

Some days I feel like I have earned a black belt in staying centered, meaning that I have a well-developed practice of finding and resetting the calm in my center in response to the challenge of my day or mothering tasks. Seeing this as a daily practice is a proactive way of engaging the mothering load. Below are some essential aspects of this mothering practice.

1. *Walk away and breathe*: Move away from stressful energy and take in some fresh inspiration.

2. *Say blessings*: Blessings align the energy field and call helpful energies to us. Perhaps this is where the "praying mother" stereotype comes from, but try it and see how gently effective it is.

3. *Lie down on the earth or the couch*: If weather permits, lying directly on the earth is best, but the couch will do as well. Taking a few minutes to set down your burdens and rest is a powerful way to reboot. Imagine releasing your stress down into the ground, and then notice and receive the new energy potential available in this moment.

4. *Take a walk*: Get your body and your children moving. A walk does wonders for rejuvenating the body and soul. Even

better, bring your children to a wild place and replenish yourselves through direct contact with Mother Nature.

5. *Make some structural repairs*: Identify where the overall structure is not working. Do you need a babysitter, self-care, early bedtimes, a date, a family meeting? Are kids overtired, stressed, over-scheduled, in a new developmental phase, in need of bodywork? Do you all need more quality time together?

6. *Plan something fun*: Call a friend for a play date, bake a tasty treat, watch a movie, turn on some music and dance—switch the energy from stress by changing your focus to fun.

7. *Open your heart*: First of all, open it to yourself by breathing into your heart center. Mothering as a spiritual path is exquisitely challenging at times. Remember the imperfection of it all and that you are not required to fix it. Every moment can be a fresh start when you come from the powerful energy of the heart.

Key Energy Meditations

In my practice of mothering from the center, I have developed some key meditations. This practice does not mean that I remain in a Zen state no matter how rowdy my children are; rather, it is a practice of aligning the overall energy and guiding them in caretaking their own energy. To work with energy, I typically use my inner vision to "see" energy like streams of light, sense it like a rush of coolness or warmth, and breathe toward an intended place while sending energy along with the breath. Here are some specific applications:

• *Birth energy and soul talks.* One of the main energy tools I use is connecting, from my own center, with the birth energy of each of my children. I may see them with my mind's eye or sense their energy. The birth energy flow is a powerful point of connection that serves your child for life and sustains your mothering. Strengthen this potential by sending a breath from your center to your child, breathing the life-force energy to them. From this meditative space, have a soul talk with your child by asking how he or she is doing or what he or she needs.

• *Calming the energy and soothing conflicts.* When someone in the family is out of balance in his or her energy or a conflict is arising, practice sensing the energy from your own center. You may say a blessing, send birth energy to your child, or engage him or her directly with touch or guidance, depending on the sense you receive from your center. Become quiet and drop into pure presence. Focus on each child's energy field and ask for the insight needed to address any imbalances. Listen from this center point when a child is expressing sadness or other emotions so you can hear his or her true feelings and needs.

• *Soothing conflicts with a specific child.* If you are experiencing conflict repeatedly with a child, again, tune in to the birth energy flow. Call to mind the alignment of his or her birth field and breathe this energy toward the child to rebalance your energies. You may do this as a meditation or while touching or holding your child, and notice how working with your energy connection facilitates a greater ease between you. Rather than trying to solve conflict directly, begin with rebalancing the energy by attuning to your own center and receiving insight or guidance from there. When conflict is routine with a child, it is also helpful to find external support from an experienced mother/friend, bodyworker, teacher, or counselor. Every child is a blessing, but when this blessing is elusive, it is time to call upon more resources. Maintain focus on the blessing of this child and then seek the assistance to receive it.

- *Clearing disruptive energy.* When someone is repeatedly cranky, I recommend making a spiritual bath (page 13) to clear the whole house and everyone's energy field. You may invite your child to make the spiritual bath with you. Your child will often be cheerful or at ease by the time you finish making the bath, having cleared the stagnancy in his or her energy.

- *Tending a sick child.* Our bodies have healing energy for our child just with our presence, particularly if we can let go of fear and open to the love we have for our children. Stay near your sick child and release every to-do item. Rest and read, blessing your child with your calm presence in the quiet spaciousness; both of you will emerge from the illness feeling replenished. Injuries can also be supported with presence when you allow a child to cry and release emotional energy while simply holding him or her in your arms.

- *Transforming worry to blessing energy.* As a parent, there are countless opportunities to worry, but worry disrupts the flow in the energy field. When you feel worried about a child for any reason, breathe your worry down into the earth and then turn it into a blessing for them, countering the worry and restoring energy alignment. For example, a worry about children leaving may become a blessing: *May they be protected while they are away from home.* Or for illness: *May their body be strong and restored to health.* Once you clarify the energy, you can also more clearly receive intuition that is valid and essential for protecting your child. Differentiate a protective intuition from fear or unfounded worry by connecting to your center. Intuition has a solid and unwavering quality, whereas fear or worry feels contracted and dissipates with breath in the center. Listen to and follow through on your protective instincts for your child.

- *Increasing joy and gratitude.* The quality of energy around us is enhanced in the presence of joy, love, and gratitude. Playing with children, snuggling together, giving hugs, sensing the love for one another, and encouraging family members to express gratitude—all are powerful energy practices. My sons know the phrase "Find a grateful heart, please," which is what I say when I am encouraging them to remember their gratitude. Also, blessing the house and each child with words or a spiritual bath increases the radiance and potential for nourishment, as does focusing on the moments of gratitude in each day as a mother, even when not feeling especially grateful.

- *Envisioning the potential.* I do a centering meditation every morning for about four minutes while drinking a cup of tea. During this time I envision, and thus energize, the potential of the day and our family. In my inner mind, I might "see" the family engaging happily together, sense the quality of this particular day, ask for guidance and extra support, or set an intention for myself as a creative being. The body will magnify what we hold in the center, and we can be intentional about the potential we cultivate.

- *Instant refresh.* Engage this practice whenever you need to instantly refresh the energy around you. Look out the window or imagine yourself in nature, and exhale every stress or burden you have been carrying. Next, inhale the beauty of the earth and invite it to replenish your cells and energy field. Repeat for three to nine breath cycles. Stepping outside into the fresh air or placing bare feet onto the earth can also clear the energy (for you or your children). Having cleared the dense energy of the challenge or frustration that adds to your mothering load, return to your work or mothering with this new potential around you. Teach this exercise to your older children when homework or other stresses feel overwhelming to them.

- *Calming the dragon.* My eight-year-old son invented this exercise. One day, he noticed my stress and anger increasing in the presence of several mothering frustrations. He held up a small dragon statue and said, "Mom, how about if I hold this up when you are getting angry, so you can stop." It was so simple—and it worked. When the steam was rising out of my center, my children would run to find the dragon statue. Seeing the statue in front of me often made me laugh, or at least helped me remember that I had a choice in my energy response. Sometimes I call to mind the dragon statue on my own as a reminder to recalibrate myself in any given moment.

• *Directing the flow.* My children often hear energetic directions like "Find your center," "Keep your energy in your own space," "Notice what is happening in your energy," or "Please calm your energy." I have them close their eyes and locate the inner space in their body to sense their own energy. I ask them to feel the energy connection between us, as well as to understand how it feels when their energy is out of balance or how it might align to support the overall family flow. I also invite them to select an area of the house to tend for ten to fifteen minutes. Tending the home or doing other activities together restores the harmonic flow.

Often, when a conflict arises, one child has his energy over in the field of the other. Again, I teach them to sense their own center and return their energy to this personal energy field. I practiced this skill with my oldest son, inviting him to direct his energy toward me and then bring it back to his own center as he sat behind me. I would say "now" every time I felt his energy in my space and "back" when it was back in his space.

My son was amazed that I could tell the difference in the direction of his energy, but we can all sense energy if we practice. He said to me, "Now what does it feel like?"

I answered, "It feels like you're choking me."

He answered, "Yes! I was imagining having my hands around your neck."

"Great, honey. That's lovely," I responded sarcastically.

He wanted to continue. "Now what do you feel?"

I sensed his energy from my center and said, "It feels like flowing water."

"Wow, Mom," he said in awe. "I was imagining myself surfing. That is so cool."

That is the power of energy medicine.

Milky Season and Transitions in Mothering

I loaded three bags of well-worn toys and faded and outgrown clothing into the car in a ritual that I make two to three times a year to pare down the clutter that seems to incessantly accumulate in our household. At the last minute, I pulled out a pair of running shoes that were still almost new, worn for a month after their purchase, and then—with subsequent pregnancies and postpartum periods—left to sit in my closet while my primary exercise came from birthing, lifting, and carrying my first, then second, and now third child. But the kids were getting older, and maybe I would go for a run sometime. I decided to pull them out of the giveaway bag, though my tired body was not so sure.

A decade of parenting can pass so quickly. Sometimes I stop myself and just watch the boys, to take in the moment. My oldest son is becoming more self-aware, though. The other day, he noticed me looking at him and said, "What?"

I smiled in return but thought, *I'm pondering your radiance while you are still here in front of me, before you slip away into your own life.*

My children have invited me into so many new adventures, including swords and shields; Legos; soccer; children's bodywork;

new friendships; playground adventures; and a multitude of songs, stories, and games. We have navigated conflicts; adopted two parrots; learned to swim; played guitar; and added four guitars, two ukuleles, and a piano to our living room. We have gone through preschool, grade school, middle school, and all the rituals and events each grade or year includes. And through it all, I have borne witness to the unfolding of each unique soul as my children have interacted, in ever-expanding context, with the world.

Each change for the boys has invited a change in work structures or family rhythms. For a decade, I worked primarily on Saturdays, with my husband then at home to accommodate the needs of our young children. As they moved further into the realm of busy weeks full of school and activities, we realized that this work schedule needed to shift to allow for more family time on the weekends.

Some of these changes are clear markers on the passage of time. Like the summer that our youngest son stopped nursing, became fully potty-trained, and started preschool. The last traces of babyhood fell away, which marked a major family shift as well. We moved out the changing table—an item that had been a staple in our bedroom—and my son and I had some gentle talks about it being time to stop nursing, or "having milkies." Though he was having his "milkies" only occasionally at that point, nursing was a big comfort to the little guy.

My own body had given all it could with a decade of pregnancy and nursing; it was time to make the transition. Upon meeting this transition point, my son sobbed in my arms. We talked about the hugs and love that would continue to be a part of his life. Through his tears, he asked me, "Is milky season over?"

I looked into his bright eyes and said, "Yes, honey, milky season is over—for me, too." He would be the last child I would nurse.

Learning how to make transitions is essential for children. Though we would like to spare them any heartache in life, we actually enhance our bond and their life skills when we stay with them while they meet the grief, anxiety, and excitement of a transition. Each time we support our children in making a transition—to their own bed, to a new grade level or school, to spending a night away, and so on—we teach them valuable skills for meeting the changes that accompany life.

That fall, after we stopped nursing, he began preschool in our neighborhood at a lovely program taught by a master teacher named Mia. Being naturally social and a gardener at heart, he happily made new friends and played in the outdoor garden. Mia shared with me that one day, when the children gathered around the last few blueberries on a bush in the yard, she told them that this was the last of the blueberries for the year. My son came to her and softly whispered, "Blueberry season is over, and milky season is over."

Perhaps on that same morning, I slipped on the running shoes that I had pulled from the bag. I put them on my feet and hopped up and down. They felt springy, and I felt light wearing them. With all my children in school for the first time, I went for a run. I ran toward the park. My joints were stiff, and I had to alternate between walking and running. Still, the autumn light was spilling all around me, and I ran faster than I had in so many years of holding little hands and pushing strollers. Then the tears came. I did not even know I had tears to cry. But they came and spilled down my cheeks. Milky season was over, and another season soon would come.

Meeting Grief as a Part of Transitions

After I stopped nursing, I noticed that my body felt less supple. Without oxytocin, the feel-good hormone of breastfeeding, my nerves were more brittle, too. While nursing, my breasts were full and round with milk. I adored my milk-laden breasts. There is nothing more feminine than the gentle curves of the female body.

And I enjoyed nursing. There is a true bodily satisfaction in holding a baby and watching the milk-inspired expressions while he or she drinks from the breast, eyes half-closed, the softness of baby lips meeting the softness of the nipple.

But then the oxytocin stopped. Suddenly I was snapping at everyone. It was as if I had awakened from a peaceful slumber. Those nursing hormones had softened the edges of my boys' arguing and daily demands. Now everything felt harsh and sharp. To top off these new irritations, I found that, beyond the softness of babies, milk-filled breasts, and nursing, my breasts had changed shape and my worn-out bra kept sliding up.

It is said that *change is the only constant*. How many times had I been through this as a mother—my body changing with each pregnancy and birth; the expansion and contraction that accompanies each child's entry; the transformation of myself as a woman, sharing my body and life with my children; the transition in a relationship as it moves from partners to parents; the rapidly evolving beings themselves as they embody the womb, come into being, and then begin walking around with distinct desires of their own. Now there I was again, coming back to my body, transformed to a new and different form.

I felt grief. What I know about grief is that it is a normal part of letting go of an old form. Too often we try to make ourselves feel better by skipping the natural process of grieving that actually helps us make the transition to a new place. So I cried. I talked with my husband and friends. I acknowledged the complex emotions in my center, coming to terms with another set of changes. I felt what was there and then I released it with each tear, word spoken, and internal acknowledgment.

Once grief is released, the movement to restore life begins. I began to clear my closet and drawers of every ill-fitting bra or loose shirt that no longer felt good on my body. I went shopping and purchased some new clothing. I noticed that I was drawn to bright shades of pink mixed with gray, bold patterns, ruffles, and layered tank tops. At each evolution of our children, we may evolve as well. With my new form came the next phase of expression for my creative self.

Love is the most powerful energy current. My breasts had nourished three beautiful boys and provided a tenderness that would buffer them in this world. Now I returned the favor. I caressed my breasts, each one resting perfectly in my palms, and I gave thanks for them and all they had given. I called to mind the words of my youngest son who, long after he stopped nursing, would say, "Tell the milkies I love them."

What transitions have you made on your mothering journey? How have you or your family been transformed?

Cycles of Ease and Challenge

Families have cycles of ease or challenge, depending on the changes occurring for each member of the family. In families with multiple children, one child can be in a place of ease while another is showing the stress of learning or integrating new skills. Navigating the periods of ease and challenge among each family member adds additional complexity. Take note of the ease—the smiling baby, the curious toddler, the passions of children and teens—and add buffers, such as rest and play, for the challenges. Likewise, major transitions may require more time or support than expected. When shifting from the routine of school to the more open nature of summer, it can take several weeks for children—and the family—to adjust. My children are often crankier, more emotional, and have more conflicts or complaints during these times, revealing the stress they are feeling. The transition back to school causes the same issues, so I schedule a lighter workload for myself in order to be more available to support this process.

With a first baby, your life re-forms around that one child. But if you add a second or third child or more, everyone in the family has to recalibrate. When my third baby was three months old, I took him and my four-year-old son on a hike with a friend. I expected a peaceful outing, but my older son repeatedly resisted any request to stay close on the scenic but precarious trail. At one point, he scrambled to the top of a tall, sheer rock, ignoring my commands to stop. With my infant in a sling, I was not able to follow him with the quick reaction that was needed; within seconds, he was far beyond my grasp. I untied the sling, passed the baby to my friend, and then scrambled up to the dizzying height where my young son sat laughing. I was stressed, worried, and even embarrassed that my son was not listening to me.

Now, in hindsight, I can appreciate the developmental changes that occur around three and four years of age and cause children to test boundaries. I also appreciate how those changes coincided with the internal conflict and emotions for a child whose mother's attention was now devoted to the intensive care of a newborn. Mothers in a similar situation, with a toddler or preschool-age child and a baby, will find themselves challenged and likely exhausted by balancing this dynamic. During my own experiences of straddling the needs of multiple young children, I often called upon spirit as divine intervention in order to find more patience. I learned that it was essential to have plenty of rest and keep our days simple. When my third son turned four years old, it was my first time parenting a child this age without a baby. I found that my son still tested the boundaries, but in the absence of newborn caretaking demands and sleep deprivation, I had much deeper reserves to meet him.

Making Time and Space for Transitions
Transitions will always take longer for children to integrate than adults. Expect several weeks or even months for a child to acclimate

to a new routine. Add more structure, like childcare, play dates, and downtime, to ease periods of stress or transition. Recognize that stress responses are a natural process of transition and skill building. If you suspect that a child is working on new skill levels or transitioning into a new developmental age, it is helpful to increase your patience and just listen to (rather than attempt to solve) their frustrations. They may simply need an outlet for emotional expression during these times. Make space for yourself during transitions as well. Buffers in your schedule will ease your stress and give room for you to process the change. Slow your pace and invite spaciousness in order to be present and bear witness to the essential, like a passage from preschool to kindergarten or other profound milestones.

If a fundamental change is occurring, such as a major move, a separation or divorce, or an illness or emergency, it is essential to bring in major support. Make time for connecting, reassuring, and playing with your children. Call upon trusted family members and friends. Resist the urge to explain the details of what is happening to your children, no matter how mature they might seem. Children deserve to stay in the more carefree zone of childhood as much as is possible. Enlist a counselor trained in working with children to help them sort through emotional stress, because children do not typically process their feelings by talking. In fact, talking too much can add to their stress level.

Support an aligned flow in the family by using energy tools, incorporating blessings, providing extra hugs, and doing the activities that increase everyone's laughter and joy. Laughter moves energy and accesses the heart potential. If you have a particular challenge, bless the most difficult aspects or people involved because this is where the energy will become most congested. Likewise, in the case of divorce, it is essential to be kind and bless your former partner because your children are connected to each of you on a cellular level. Children will feel any parental discord within their own centers. Add ease to these situations by offering blessings and generating positive energy by simply laughing and hugging more frequently.

When well-loved neighbors who had been particularly playful and generous to our boys moved away, I noticed that my children were quicker to conflict or tears. Their grief at this loss was not expressed directly but rather through their emotional state. To help them acknowledge the loss, I said, "I think maybe you're feeling sad because our friends moved. I miss them, too." I made extra attempts to play with them and attend to them directly, though compared to our empty-nest neighbors who had an affinity for Legos and rocket building, I knew I was a poor substitute. However, I could offer my steady presence. Love grows from being together in the difficulties as well as the joys.

As the anchor for the family, make sure that you and your partner are being nourished as individuals and as partners. If one of you encounters a rough period where your emotions are running high and your patience levels low, it is time to assess your needs. Are you having enough exercise, rest, and fun? Are you at peace with where you are and able to engage your creative essence? Is there a change happening that requires acknowledgment or support? Because of children's unpredictable needs and schedules, mothers may feel isolated or lonely. In mothering (and parenting), you are doing sacred work. Attending to yourself on a routine basis positions you, and the family, for long-term success.

Are you in a cycle of ease or challenge?
What ease can you savor?
What challenge requires additional support?

Being in the Beauty

One day while walking my two older sons home from school, I must have been wearing a frown because my oldest son asked, "What's wrong, Mom?"

His words jolted me back to my center. My attention was far from being with my boys. I had instead been contemplating a series of things that needed to be done.

"Oh, nothing's wrong, honey," I replied. "I'm just a little overwhelmed with what I need to do today."

He turned to me and said, "How about if you just kick me?"

"Kick you?" I responded with alarm. "Why would I kick you?"

He said, "That's how I get my frustrations out. Here, watch." He called to his brother, "Hey, Gabe! Kick me!"

Gabe did not hesitate for a minute. He ran straight at his brother and jumped into the air with a powerful flying kick.

I was so surprised by the whole exchange that I began to laugh. My energy was instantly lighter just from witnessing my boys in action.

"See, Mom? It works!" he yelled, running ahead with his brother.

Yes, honey, I see. I see your beauty again and again. This is my invitation as mother.

EIGHT

Healing the Mothering Heart

In Chinese medicine, the womb is considered a second heart. One of the first signs of pregnancy is the baby's heartbeat within the womb. The heart has the most powerful energy field in the body, and it begins beating for each one of us in our mother's womb. I see the mothering heart as the connection between a woman's heart and her womb, the two potent places in the female body. The combined energies of the heart and womb allow a mother to create a powerful field of love for nurturing herself and her creations, even across space and time. To access this energetic capacity more fully, we must heal the mothering heart. Children call us to the center of ourselves, and they also invite the healing of the heart-womb connection.

When I gave birth to my second son, I also was laboring on a creative project. My first book had found its way to a prominent

New York City literary agent in the mind-body-spirit genre. Though we met midway through my pregnancy, the book project went out to a large group of publishers the day I went into labor. Later I would wonder if this dual laboring caused some of the interference pattern that seemed to prolong my son's birth process. It felt like I was laboring twins. Our creative essence is connected to all the soulful creations we make, and so it was that I labored the energy of birth for both my baby and my book on the same night.

After the labor, my newborn child found himself welcomed into our home. My book, however, was turned down by the major publishing houses in New York. My literary agent was so known and trusted that he expected the project to move forward with ease. *The Vagina Monologues*, by Eve Ensler, had been hugely successful in New York and around the country, creating new dialogue around the female body. My agent had hand-selected women at every major publishing house in New York to receive my book about the sacred energy of the pelvic bowl (which would serve as the inspiration for the later published *Wild Feminine*).

Not only did the female publishing executives universally reject the book, but they also were quite uncomfortable with the content and with the notion of the pelvic bowl as having energy or being sacred. For me, that collective response was shocking. Having just traveled to the spirit door myself to birth my baby, I was immersed in the birth field and sacred birth flow. I could not comprehend this reality: We had come so far in our professional opportunities as women, and yet we had lost the connection to our essential feminine nature. How could we repair this separation when women—my own gender, some of whom held the keys to the publishing world— had internalized patterns of patriarchy and so completely forgotten their own sacred origins and this potential in their bodies?

I rocked my new baby, inhaling the scent of his downy hair and soft skin, and cried. I told him, "I'm so glad you are here, on the other side. And I'm very sad right now. I'm so glad for your entry, and sad to see how the culture has forgotten that this entry is sacred."

He slept deeply and peacefully in my arms; it was a home, after all, that would honor his sacredness.

Repairing the Spirit-Body Divide

Several months later, I would contact a few of the smaller spiritually focused publishers. One by one, they told me the same thing: we work with spiritual material but not in regard to "that part" (the vagina and pelvic bowl) of the body. I was referred to presses with a feminist orientation. The feminist presses liked the how-to content for attending to the female body but did not want any "woo-woo" or spiritual material.

Now I could see clearly: The divide between spirit or the sacred and a woman's body was so vast that even our structures embodied this bifurcation. The publishing realm could receive a book about the female body or a book of spirit but not one that linked the two. The people who created these companies and then ran them embodied this separation between body and spirit as well. This is also why mothers often feel invalidated, because the sacredness of their work is unrecognized and unrecognizable. Though my book was intended to bridge this divide, the fracture needed far more repair than I had realized. The knowledge weighed heavily on my mothering heart.

By mothering from the center, I have learned to look for the energy within myself whenever the external world is not providing what I seek. So I went into my center and my mothering realm to receive the guidance and direction from the deeper currents. In the early spring after my second baby's birth, I took both my children to a wild place near our home. I cried out to spirit, *What can I do with this split between the sacred and the body? How will we heal? How can I tell my children to follow their dreams? How will I teach them they are sacred when the world will tell them otherwise?*

We were sitting at the river's edge when the water began to drum against the riverbank. My older son said, "Mama, the water is talking to us."

I answered, "I know—but I have no idea what it's saying."

Just then an eagle flew past our place in the sand, low along the edge of the river, almost near enough to touch. I felt an instant peace, as if all I had asked had been answered. It was an answer from spirit, but even more, it was a reconnection through my mothering body to that of divine source. Though it would take time to discover, I now had the energy current in place to continue my journey.

My experience at the river inspired my purchase of a Native American hand drum. I began a practice of drumming with my children. At the river's edge or the ocean, I made a fire with sticks that we gathered and played the drum while they dug in the sand. In returning to the wild and drumming, I expanded my own energy potential to the greater realm of spirit. Intentionally forging this connection to spirit, I was more than myself in these times. In the divine flow I could replenish my energy field, receive visions to guide our family and my work, and ask for the blessings needed to heal my mothering heart. The renewed access to spirit within my own center provided guidance for another way.

Resolving a Painful Lineage

In one of my workshops for women, I relay the story of our maternal lineage with a series of small bowls that fit one inside another. This placing of the bowls illustrates the womb of each woman held by her mother and then, in turn, carried her child. As such, our wombs are energetically linked across time. They contain the imprints of our lineage, both the helpful and painful.

One day as I was placing a set of tiny clay bowls to make my point, I stood to explain this energy potential of our lineage. Forgetting that I had lined the bowls across the floor, I stepped back in my excitement and crushed one of the bowls under my foot. It was the largest bowl but just the size of a silver dollar, and I had suggested that it represented my great-great-grandmother. The roomful of women gasped all at once. It was as if I had crushed the soul of my long-lost maternal ancestor. A shock passed through me as well. I reached down to tenderly recover the pieces of "her bowl." They were large enough that I would be able to glue them back together, as I reassured myself and the women watching me carefully.

I pondered this woman, the great-great-grandmother of my maternal line. The only thing I knew of her was that she had a breakdown of some sort and left her family of five children, one of whom was my great-grandmother, Nana. In effect, the crushing of this woman's bowl seemed symbolic of her own actions in renouncing her role as mother. Though I do not know what led her to this extreme action, there is a fierce understanding among the women who came after her: *As a mother, you do not leave your children.*

After gluing the clay bowl back together, the lines of the fracture defined the shape. Now it looked distinctly like a rose. Though the wounds of a lineage make imprints, how we hold the imprints is up to us. We can ponder what we have received and what we would like to change. Working with the energy of our own center, we can always make a rose.

Wounding patterns in a lineage, a painful relationship with your mother or father, or a difficult childhood—all can leave imprints in your energy field. Even if these childhood imprints and wounds are dormant, they still affect how openly you meet the world. Resolving these painful imprints is a step-by-step process in that you often embody the limiting patterns or the reactions to them yourself.

The presence of your children will bring these lineage patterns to the surface, making them more visible but also more accessible to change. That means that if you were neglected as a child, you will find challenge in being present with your own child. If there were patterns of scarcity, then you will have difficulty accessing your potential for abundance. Or if there was anger in your household as a child, you will likely meet your own anger, and the unmet needs it signals, as a mother. This is true with fear and other emotions. Whatever was in the house of your childhood, you can expect to encounter these patterns in your body. Even though you want to parent differently, having the intention is not enough. You have to change the core patterns and imprinted framework that organize your life energy.

The Mothering Edge and Opportunities to Heal

Healing or changing the imprints that give form to creative flow means working at your mothering edge. This is your boundary or capacity for remaining centered in a potent field of life-enhancing energy, rather than contracting into a reaction pattern that produces a stagnant core. In changing these imprints, it is not helpful to be in denial about the patterns you carry or judge yourself and feel guilty when you succumb to a toxic reaction or mother in less-than-ideal ways. Again, the stresses in raising children are real, and the many factors and emotions that mothers and parents have to balance are routinely overwhelming. However, in this intensity, there is also tremendous opportunity to address those (otherwise hidden) limiting beliefs and unmet needs.

Nurturing your mothering soul, especially in the most difficult moments, will free your creative energy and allow it to move as a vibrant current in your body and life. This process entails slowing down your interactions with your children, particularly the highly emotional exchanges, to examine the energy beneath them. For example, when you begin having a strong reaction in the center of your body to a crying baby, the challenging behaviors of a three-year-old, or a moody teenager, rather than engaging your child with an emotional response (particularly a highly charged or off-center one), step away from the encounter.

Find the ground beneath you and notice what is happening to your body and energy field. Notice the sensations within and the emotions they contain. You may invite calm by just simply witnessing yourself. Breathe energy down toward the earth. Ask yourself what you need and how you can meet at least one simple need right now, whether it's taking a breath, lying down for a moment, stepping outside, making contact with another adult, or saying a blessing to spirit. Likely your past wounds are rising to the surface in the stress of your mothering. Meeting one need, or even letting the light of spirit touch your center, brings healing. To change the lineage imprint, focus on your desires rather than on what was missing. Let yourself feel this edge of the new potential, which, like birth, can be uncomfortable as you stretch your range of expression or forge a new way of being.

Doing this day by day, one situation at a time, radically shifts the patterns of your core, allowing peace and connection even in the midst of stress or conflict. It invites a vibration of love in the previous place of raw anger or scarcity. Though it is work, the rewards are immense. As you heal, the energy required to protect old wounds or guard the heart is liberated for more creative pursuits. In providing for your children what was missing for you, you have the opportunity to be remade and to rediscover the sensations of delight that come with your birthright of joyful embodiment.

Women's Stories:
Replacing Shame with the Power of Potential

As the mother of a four-year-old boy and a new baby girl, Shannon came for pelvic work to heal the effects of two vaginal births and to understand more about the potential in her center for mothering. While I was working to relieve the tension of her left pelvis, I asked how she was doing in the transition to two children. Tears immediately formed in her eyes as she shared her difficulties.

Shannon related that she found herself increasingly embarrassed by the rough play of her son with other children and his growing fascination with weapons and destruction. She did not want his play to offend the other mothers whose children were in her son's playgroup and felt awkward in her attempts to address his behavior. He also had major tantrums, when his screams echoed through the house. As a self-defined "pleaser," Shannon made great efforts to take care of others, and she was increasingly ashamed of her son and his behavior. She also felt less connected when shame arose.

Most mothers will face patterns of shame in raising their children, feeling inadequate in the face of mothering tasks or ashamed by certain ways their children behave. When shame arises in mothering, it reveals where we ourselves feel pressure to be perfect and to have our children reflect that perfection. We may believe that otherwise our worth is questionable, rather than knowing our value as an inherent truth. The antidote, instead of focusing on the child or their behavior, is to reclaim ourselves as sacred in place of the shame.

As Shannon spoke about her son, I directed her awareness to the response in her body. Her energy moved primarily towards her head, while her chest and pelvis contracted. Her body revealed a pattern of stress and congestion. I led her through a meditation to restore a connection to her creative center. We worked to clear the congestion and shame, blessing her core body to receive the sacred medicine it contained. Many tears flowed as she shed the restrictive energy patterns hampering her ability to grow with her child. The truth is that mothering offers a lifetime of opportunities to expand our potential if we are willing to be vulnerable and acknowledge that we do not have to be perfect or know exactly what to do or say; rather, we can ask and receive the divine assistance that is always there for us, especially in the face of our vulnerability or uncertainty.

For Shannon, the next steps included working with emotional energy in her son, understanding the energy impulses in boys, and tapping into bodywork resources to support her son's ability to more easily regulate his sensory system. But the greatest change for Shannon happened when she opened to the potential and the connection to spirit right in her own center.

After clearing the energy of her pelvic bowl, Shannon saw an image of her son. He was playing as a forest fairy, like he did when they went to the woods. She recognized how the masculine energy arising in her son could protect this fairy (or feminine) essence for him. After the meditation, she now had creative ideas for being with her son as he explored new facets of himself, whether as a fairy or a warrior. She planned to share her vision of protection. She would tell him that she understood his need to protect himself and that fairies also have ways of protecting themselves, like golden light and magic. The shame had cleared, and Shannon discovered the pure potential that arose in its place.

Receiving Support from the Great Mother

Imprints and emotions from the past pain of childhood may be stirred while mothering our own children. When a woman had a challenging relationship with her mother, becoming a mother herself can add stress, as the strain of the mother-child relationship is imprinted in her energy field. She may hope that her relationship with her child is better than her own experience with her parents.

But she will also worry and perceive the relationship through a wounded perspective, and the normal relationship stresses that occur between herself and her child may carry more emotional weight than necessary.

One of my clients, who had long-term conflict with her mother, felt that her baby was "rejecting her" when her baby kept pulling off the nipple during breastfeeding and seemed unable to make a good latch. A client without this same wounding had a similar problem but saw the breastfeeding issue in a more neutral and holistic perspective. Instead of finding emotional meaning in the situation, she sought cranial work for her baby, addressed the birth flow, and increased her rest to restore the nursing pattern from many angles. As mothers, we tend to see our children through any wounds we carry. Having awareness of this tendency is the first step in finding clarity and transformation.

Among my clients who have a strained mothering relationship, a common pattern I have noticed is that they hesitate to step into the generally left-sided aspect of their pelvic bowl, which is where most women imprint their mother's energy. It is as if they pull back from the mothering essence to avoid the pain or difficult connection there. This tendency for holding back limits their ability to actually change or address the imprint pattern, because the holding pattern requires significant energy.

A woman must step fully into the left pelvis and energy field, as this is the first step in claiming her creative space and changing the core mothering imprint. As an adult, she can create an entirely new pattern for herself and receive the mothering support that was missing. In this way, she heals the energy wound and expands her own potential. Instead of stepping around the limitations to form a mothering pattern, she can draw from her full creative capacity.

I teach women to call on the Great Mother, present in the earth's energy, to fill in the energy holes where they lacked mothering. When lying on the earth or sitting against an ancient tree, this gentle mothering presence is palpable. This is the energy that will hold us when we find that we are missing some essential ingredients for our ability to mother; instead of managing with less, we can draw this energy to our center and gain a new potential. We can ease the pain of our fathering wounds as well. Healing this mothering imprint enables us to replenish what was needed and then access our capacity in abundance rather than scarcity.

The needs of children can seem infinite, and tapping into the Great Mother essence allows us to be fed while mothering our children. When one of my children asks for something or climbs onto my lap, rather than feel as if he is taking energy from me, I use his request as a cue to expand my energy field toward spirit. In this way, we both receive replenishment from the Great Mother. I am held even as I hold another.

Exercise: The Great Mother and Expanding Your Mothering Imprints

1. Begin by lying on the earth, leaning against a tree, or sitting near a window and sensing into the vast earth and Great Mother presence. Notice the way this presence meets and responds to you. Let yourself lean into this strong kindness. Imagine setting down all your mothering or other burdens.

2. Let yourself be held; receive the support of this energy. Invite the Great Mother presence to fill and renew your whole energy field. Receive this inspiration and nurturance; let your deepest needs be met.

3. Focus on a specific desire or intention for yourself, whether it is feeling valuable, being witnessed, feeling whole, or accessing

joy, and place this into the presence of the Great Mother. Ask for her to fill this need and for you to be able to receive what you are asking for.

4. Focus on a specific desire for your mothering, whether it is having peace in the center, being able to cook or caretake with ease, to release all stress and guilt—whatever you most need, ask for it to be taken care of. Again, call upon the Great Mother. Let her energy come to you now and in the approaching days.

5. Bless yourself: *I receive the healing presence of the Great Mother into my energy field to heal and expand my mothering imprints.* May you remember the comfort of the Great Mother; call to her and receive her touch.

Restoring Your Full Creative Range

Every mother, in the act of mothering, will find her wounds, energy holes, hidden emotional sensitivities, and long-stored emotions. Like a true spiritual path, the intensity of mothering brings to light the places that restrict the radiance of your soul expression. Working with these wounded places will ultimately offer more access to your whole creative range. This means addressing your intolerance for disorder or stress, tendencies to try to control your environment, or emotional congestion points of held fear, rage, grief, and shame to reaccess your full potential. Your children will help you find your way, especially when you follow their lead.

Mothering promises to teach you how to joyfully embody your creative center, but first you may have to encounter the wounds that disassociated you from your body and pure being in the first place. Let the Great Mother hold you, and learn from the mothers in your midst. Play with your children and remember the joy of movement and sensation just as they are newly discovering the world around them. Follow their joy and notice where you hold yourself back. Invite a blessing for yourself and then continue to follow them.

Ritual is powerful medicine for reclaiming your creative center and restoring your wholeness. (*Wild Feminine* contains many ritual exercises.) Particularly when mothering is difficult or you do not know what is needed in a given situation, access the energy currents that interface with spirit through ritual. Ritual can be as simple as engaging with the elements of earth, fire, water, and air and calling to the greater realm of spirit. Sit on the earth and be held. Make a spiritual bath with garden herbs. Wash your face with the dew from a plant. Let a breeze smooth your energy field. Create a ritual for your family. I like to make a fire ritual with one of my girlfriends by placing papers containing both the words of our grief and blessings into the fire and offering them to spirit. You can heal core layers by allowing spirit to touch you and in the process create new ways of being for yourself.

How is mothering inviting you to heal?

Where do you need more support to continue your transformation?

How does attending to the energy in your center change your mothering or bring healing?

Past Abuse and Other Profound Wounds

A person may not encounter the full emotional impact of past wounds until they become a parent. Memories that were previously dormant may surface in the process of parenting. When trauma from the past arises along with the stress of taking care of a child, it can be a volatile combination.

If you are overwhelmed by emotional burdens of past pain, work with those who can support you in making an entirely new emotional and energetic framework. Recognize when you are unable to find equilibrium on your own and seek professional help. Addressing the profound wounds of physical, emotional, or sexual abuse that have roots in your past family patterns requires skilled support to heal fully. Cherish yourself and your mothering enough to receive this support; you need not be alone in your pain. Prepare for a long-term process of healing that will pay dividends for your health and the health of your children.

Working with Hitting Energy and Anger

If a woman was hit as a child or if she witnessed physical violence, she will have the imprint of hitting energy in her field that may be triggered in the presence of stress and anger. Since parenting is a highly stressful venture—with lack of sleep, hormonal shifts, babies crying, children having tantrums, and endless caregiving demands—resisting an impulse to hit in response to stress can be quite challenging until the imprint is healed.

It is typically necessary to work with a skilled counselor to fully change this pattern, but addressing your own energy response is also helpful. When stress triggers your body's impulse to hit, strike out, or even be harsh with yourself, fold your body onto the ground to give the energy a place to go. Ideally, you need to ground the energy—to literally send it down into the earth rather than follow the impulse to rage or lash out. When you are successful in grounding the energy, your body will relax and your breathing will soften. You may feel heat or energy move from your body toward the earth; let it go, and set down the burdens you have carried this far. Underneath the rage you may find grief and many unmet needs. Let it all go. You will ultimately be more free to create a bountiful life.

Sometimes it is necessary to remove yourself from the source of stress, such as a crying child, and go into another room. Placing a pillow over your head or stepping into the bath can also be helpful. These hitting energy imprints are like lightning bolts. Grounding the energy will teach your body a new pattern; instead of following the energy impulse, you move toward the ground. In the presence of stress, it is normal to have tension in the body but not to hurt others or yourself. Grounding the energy over time will teach you to manage the stress response so that it is more contained and less activating.

As your nervous system heals and learns how to deal with stress more effectively, it is also helpful to limit overall stress. Keep your commitments minimal, ask for extra help, take breaks from your children, get plenty of sleep, limit your intake of caffeine or substances that increase your body's stress level, and put into place practices that help you relax or recharge your energy. Being able to stay in your own center, rather than simply tuning in to the stress of the environment around you, is part of establishing a sense of calm in the midst of any chaos.

Anger or rage rise from your unmet needs—and even those unmet needs of your lineage. Unconsciously you may believe that your needs cannot or will not be met. Ironically, raging about the situation may push away your partner and the very help you need. Attend to yourself and establish an internal radar that alerts you to your needs early on, before stress overloads your system. Needs can be met with peace in your center by putting new patterns into practice. When you move from a calm and centered place, you are more likely to know what your needs are and then find support for having them met. Marshall Rosenberg's book *Nonviolent Communication: A Language of Life* and its related practice are valuable resources for learning how to identify and voice your needs and how to foster connection and health in relationships.

Re-accessing Your Heart Energy

Our earliest wounds determine the openness of our heart and ability to trust others. Having children invites us to heal the heart and re-access its energy potential simply by being in the presence of their innocence, faith, and openhearted love. There are two ways I work with my own heart energy while mothering. The first is, while simply mothering, to intentionally soften the area around my chest and heart, breathing toward my heart center each time I embrace my baby or child. In the beginning, I realized my chest was taut, resistant, and slightly numb from protection. Over time, my heart space reawakened with each invitation to connect with these tender and loving children. Now my children and I can more readily share our heart energy with one another. Not only do children want to be loved, but they also want their parents to receive their love.

The second way I have worked with my heart energy is during times of conflict or challenge with my children, such as when they are having a tantrum. Unless our own tantrums as a child were met with compassion, we learned to close our own heart in the presence of conflict or emotional stress. Closing the heart means that we begin to operate from the head or logical place during the conflict, instead of accessing the energy of the heart. When the heart is closed, the heart center becomes more tense. This response blocks the flow of the heart, causing physical tension in the chest and restricting the breath.

When a conflict arises in your family, practice sensing and breathing into the heart space. Opening the energy flow of the heart in this way, you will notice that you approach a conflict differently. Rather than trying to fix a challenging situation with your child, simply be with what is. Keep your heart energized and access heart energy with the child in distress. This practice not only offers more resources for parenting but also reduces the stress you will feel. Breathe into your heart and remember your love for this child.

The air around you will soften in the presence of your love-filled heart, easing the way for you both.

Exercise: Envisioning a Creative Motherhood

Mothering can feel constrictive and limiting at times, whether we are in the midst of daily stresses or encountering past imprints or unconscious patterns. Overcoming these patterns that restrict us, we recognize our infinite potential to envision a creative motherhood.

1. What does mothering and even the word *mother* mean to you? How do you see yourself as a mother or creative woman? Take a moment to find an image that coveys your present state of mothering. Is this what you want to cultivate?

2. Now imagine your mothering in the context of your wild feminine landscape. There are physical tasks or ways of being that may define your mothering, but these can be infused with the energy of spirit. The greater energy field can inspire new patterns of mothering. How would you like to be inspired as a woman and a mother? Let the energy come to you and even heal past imprints of mothering.

3. Call to mind your most essential creative fire. What is it that stirs your passion? As you focus on this creative vision, notice how your energy responds. Are you making space for this fire and tending it on a regular basis? How could it energize your mothering? Every woman needs a well-tended creative fire, as everything she makes arises from this energy.

4. Set three intentions that will lead to a tangible tending of your creative fire. As you place these intentions in your creative

center, imagine how they might inspire new mothering patterns or other creative expressions.

5. Bless yourself: *May my soul expression ignite my creative motherhood.*

Restoring a Vibrant Feminine and Masculine Essence for Our Children

To access our infinite potential in mothering, we must restore a vibrant feminine and masculine essence for ourselves and our children. The true feminine is the vibrant inspiration of our left energy field—the intuitive, holistic, receptive, visionary aspect of our right brain and left body that is focused on *receptivity* and *being*. When we drop into this feminine state of being, we find an expanded potential in the pure moment, where every sensation becomes richer. We can see the beauty right in front of us and in the divine essence of our children.

The true masculine is the dynamic potential of our right energy field—the projective, focused, linear, playful aspect of our left brain and right body that is focused on *action* and *doing*. In the presence of the feminine and the inspiration that arises from her connection, the masculine does not simply "do" but instead builds soul-filled aspects of our life. In the absence of the feminine, the masculine is a relentless taskmaster, emphasizing production often to the point of depletion. Many of our current structures, from businesses and professions to healthcare, are based in the non-holistic production model that makes little or no space for the feminine. Without the feminine, life becomes uninspired and loses touch with the sacred and the soul.

The work of our time is to restore our access to the feminine and rebuild an authentic masculine. In a production-oriented culture, the masculine aspect of doing has been overemphasized for all genders and has created many work and life structures that take us away from the home and the heart of living. We have lost touch with our feminine skills of presence, nourishment, and holistic caretaking, which mothering calls us back to.

Mothering gives us the opportunity to return home and remember the inner fire of the feminine. Ideally, both women and men will learn to tend the inner feminine fires that are meant to fuel and influence our creative expression. With a vibrant feminine, our outer masculine fires become more sustainable and soul-based rather than simply producing in an endless cycle.

Just as an unbalanced masculine system emphasizes production even to the point of depletion, a woman who mothers without access to her feminine energy will caretake to the point of exhaustion. She may be routinely harsh with herself, her children, and her partner. Mothering will feel like a wearisome duty, because she lacks the inspiration and nourishment of the feminine in her own center. Energetically closed off from that which will sustain her, she must change her core patterns in order to re-form her experience of mothering.

A feminine-masculine model of mothering means that there is time for rest and pleasure alongside working or caretaking in an inspired manner. There are seasonal rhythms that alternate between active doing and restorative rest. A mother who accesses this potential will be productive but in a more sustainable way. In touch with her own center, she may conserve her chi and defer tasks or, alternately, accomplish tasks when she has the energy to do so. She will sense her children from a deeper place of the energy realm, remembering touch and imagination. Instead of fixing or doing, she can simply be with what is and receive what is needed in that moment. In the feminine flow, she can access the expanded resources of spirit for guidance, inspiration, and peace.

We restore the feminine when we make time for inner sustenance and honor the sacred and cyclical nature of our female body, which aligns with the earth. Likewise, teaching our children to respect their bodies begins with respecting our own body—in how we talk about ourselves and our body parts, our menstrual cycles, and even how we alternate between periods of activity and rest. Cherishing ourselves shows children how to cherish themselves; they learn by observing our actions. We can also use respectful words and thoughtful regard with our children through our touch, changing diapers, and toilet training, and later on when discussing puberty or sex—all as ways to honor their inherent sacredness.

We find direct access to the feminine by engaging our creative passions. Though creative pursuits may seem impractical to the logical mind, they bring a rich energy into your mothering center. By following your creative impulses and encouraging your children to do the same, you ensure a vibrant flow of the feminine in the center of your body and life. My sons are passionate about music, art, gardening, photography, carving, metal working, and cooking. Knowing the value of the feminine for them, we take classes together and seek opportunities for creative expression. Making creations with our own hands and with our children, we weave the feminine into tangible forms. In this way, the feminine will return and we can rebuild an authentic masculine—reclaiming our day-to-day ability to work with the divine.

Energy Medicine for Daughters

If you have a daughter, read *Wild Feminine* to understand the mystery of the female body. The female body has a unique and powerful energy system that is hardly understood, and most of the information I want to convey for daughters is within that book. By reading it to learn how to care for your body and work with your core creative capacity, you may pass this wisdom to your daughter so that she makes her life with her creative center as a key point of reference.

As young women prepare to menstruate, they should know the power of their blood and how it sustains the beginning of life. Teach them about natural menstrual products like cloth pads, reusable cups, or sea sponges, and generally choosing non-bleached products to attend to their bodies.

Menstruation is a time of shedding both menstrual blood and energy. It is our body's way of clearing what is no longer needed. During times of bleeding, the body's energy field is more open or permeable in order to shed excess layers. This openness is what makes a woman feel "moody," because she is more sensitive to energy during this time. She is also more intuitive and can pay attention to the intuitions she receives as guidance for herself. Because of the heightened sensitivity, this is a good time to reduce overall activity. As your daughter pays attention to her cycle, she gains a valuable tool for knowing—based on her own rhythm— when to be more internal and nurturing for herself and when to move out in the world.

If your young daughter likes to pretend she is a princess, celebrate this sparkly aspect of her self-expression. The princess is a form of the feminine and, when cherished, can be a healthy part of her relationship to the feminine. The feminine essence loves color, texture, and the radiance within all creative forms. Teach her to celebrate her inner princess—and to protect her princess with her own inner masculine knight—and you will witness a blossoming of her feminine.

Like their mothers, daughters contain the powerful doorway within, where all life begins and each one of us enters. Too often, though, they are taught to look outside themselves for validation or information. Remember your own center, as a woman, and then show your girls how to receive this essential inner guidance for everything they do and create.

Stoking the Ovarian Fire

The pelvic bowl contains the feminine and masculine fires of the left and right ovaries, respectively. The energy of the ovaries can be cultivated to enhance creative inspiration, strengthen energetic boundaries, and give form to a woman's creative essence. Teach your daughter to nourish herself by knowing what feeds her left ovary, or feminine nature. What does she love to do? The dreamy feminine is fed when we access our creative passions without concern for any specific outcome or benefit.

The right ovary, or masculine nature, is visible in the way we engage with the outer world. Is your daughter allowing her light to shine, or is she afraid of revealing her radiance? Find examples of women whose vibrant creativity can model expression for her. Support her in cultivating and sharing her talents and gifts as a way to fuel her outer fire. When her inner and outer fires are strong, she will have a better sense of her true self and be able to stand her ground.

The Female Energy Body and Finding Center

With media images and information bombarding young women in regard to their sexuality, invite daughters to close their eyes and sense the vast inner space of their bodies. Teaching them to know the essence of their female body, by sensing from within rather than looking in a mirror, reminds them that they are far more than what can be seen. This inner space is where their power lies. By turning within—for instance, as a bedtime practice (which I do with my sons as well)—they will find this still point to connect with themselves. Tell them about the purpose of their own creative energy for finding inspiration and about the power of following the lead and organization of this inner current.

As girls navigate their complex emotional relationships and focus on being accepted by peers, they can lose touch with their center. In adolescence, girls begin to formulate an identity by seeing themselves through the eyes of others (which is increasingly true among boys as well). As a mother, counter this by staying attuned to your daughter's center. Though you may worry about her as she finds her way socially, stay in touch with the truth of her soul and the birth energy that contains her inherent beauty. Reflect this potential to her as an anchor in the emotional storms by calling to mind her core energy instead of your worries. Avoid projecting your own social mishaps onto her and use blessings like *May she find those who will celebrate her beauty*. In steering your attention away from the social difficulties and back toward the light in your daughter, you will communicate, in a deep way, that an attunement with her center is more essential than attention from others. The center of the female body is a priceless resource; plant the seeds of understanding now so that she will grow to know of this precious place that contains the creative energy for her life.

Energy Medicine for Sons

In spending my days with boys, while also working intimately with the energy of the female body, I have learned about the importance of the feminine for boys. This is also where, as mothers, we are currently failing to see them. It is essential to restore the feminine aspects of mothering if we are to give our sons access to the feminine and bring forth their authentic masculine.

When my oldest son was three, he picked out a pair of pink boots at a children's store. The proprietor scooped the boots out of his hands. She whispered to me, "I'll pretend we're out of his size. I know you don't want him wearing pink boots." (I tell the full story in *Wild Feminine*.) Now my son is twelve, and it remains one of his favorite tales. Suffice it to say that I told her it was fine with me if he wore pink boots and that they actually were his size. He proudly took them back and placed them in our bag. We won some kind of battle that day but then went home and his dad asked, "Why did you let him pick out pink boots?"

Through the past decade of raising my sons, I have been shocked at the ways that the feminine brings up shame or is discouraged for boys, even by otherwise thoughtful people (including us as mothers). There is more awareness about the negative aspects of genderizing in regard to girls, but the patterns around boys are equally destructive unless we meet them directly. Because I have pioneered a Holistic Pelvic Care practice for women and write about female creative energy, people often think it is ironic that I have three boys. But to me, it is no accident. In order for boys to be seen, they need to be with people who have an intact feminine presence.

Boys Need to Be Seen

The nature of my work in the wordless realm of the physical and energetic patterns of the body has taught me to pay attention to subtleties: breath, presence, eye contact, body language. This is the realm of the feminine.

Boys and men are masters in the wordless realm. Because a touch or a gesture conveys more meaning to them than words, it is my primary mode of communication with my sons. Perhaps it was their time out in the field, as hunters, that attuned males to the more physical and less verbal mediums of communication and interpersonal exchange. Though they are adept in navigating without words, this skill is easily unrecognized because they do not (or perhaps cannot) tell us what they are experiencing.

What our sons need—and our daughters, too, of course—is to be seen. They need us to bear witness to their beauty so that they may trust and more deeply embody the essence of who they are. To be seen requires our presence, an attention not of length but of depth. A soul-to-soul meeting that says, *I see you. I know who you are. I'm glad you came.* Recognition is a form of honoring, and recognition of our children's true essence is one of the greatest gifts we can give them.

Because we are women, we often seek connection through the words we share. In attuning to words, we mothers may miss our sons' need for presence and recognition. We may also resist seeing them if we have wounding in regard to males. When one of my sons holds up, for me to see, a spaceship that he has built, he is saying, *See what I can make!* When he asks that I watch him ride up a steep hill or jump his skateboard, he is saying, *See what I can do!* When he shares a battle creature or fighting technique, he is saying, *See how strong I am!*

Though my son may be focused on an external skill or creation, he is asking me to witness him in these things. I may notice the exquisite details of what he is sharing or I may be in the midst of mothering tasks, but I do my best to give my full presence. It may be brief, but it is a meeting from my center to his that I give because I know that he needs me to bear witness to him. If I can reflect back to him the truth of his beauty, he grows in his own knowledge of himself as a whole, radiant being. In time, he owns what is rightfully his: the beauty of his own soul.

Their Emotions Run Deep and Require Support

As they enter school and beyond, boys enter a male realm that has certain codes, such as not outwardly expressing emotions or asking for help. The reaction from my thoughtful husband in regard to his son's pink boots was not from closed-mindedness but from a valid desire to protect his son from being teased. Of course, the pink boots created endless dialogue about the expression we desired for our son, but over the years I have also recognized the wisdom of acknowledging the gender codes as well as challenging their boundaries.

When my oldest son was younger and I was helping in his classroom one day, one of his girl classmates was crying. A boy classmate asked me why she was crying. I began to talk about feelings and said that she probably missed her parents. My son, sitting next to me, pressed his elbow into my arm. Confused, I continued talking about feelings, and my son elbowed me again. I stopped talking and looked at him. He clearly wanted me to be quiet. On our walk home, I asked him about it. He said, "Mom, boys don't talk about feelings like that." He was only five, and I was speechless.

Here was another gender line, self-imposed by his entering into a field of boys. This experience helped me understand the men in my life. Later, as my son felt more secure in this group of boys and gained skills to navigate the social realms, he and I would laugh about this early conversation. But still we meet these lines time and again.

On the occasions that my boys have felt the vulnerability of sadness or frustration, I have had to sit with them in the moment and help them give voice to it. Boys' emotions often go directly to anger, a primitive emotional wiring pattern that served them as hunters and warriors back when there was no time to feel the complexities of the situation.

Males also have less crossover between the two hemispheres of the brain, which means that even though they feel emotions just as deeply as females do, they may not be able to articulate what they are feeling or why. This makes them feel acutely vulnerable, and they quickly suppress the rising feeling in order to protect themselves. I give them words to identify the feeling: "I think maybe you're sad right now. It's good to let the sadness move." I use masculine words such as "I see your courage in expressing that feeling," and "You were really brave allowing your tears to flow," to encourage them in expressing their emotions. I have learned that males are far more vulnerable and emotional than I knew. And I have learned that movement, more than words, is how they discharge their emotional energy and find center.

Swords and Shields Serve a Vital Purpose

In order to access the feminine realms of emotion and intuition, boys need to be able to protect themselves. Early on with my boys, I read *Who's Calling the Shots?* a book coauthored by professor of education Nancy Carlsson-Paige, who is also the mother of actor Matt Damon. She talks about how to handle boys' war play, and the discomfort that women typically have with the swords and guns that fascinate their sons. Carlsson-Paige encourages parents and caregivers to allow boys to give expression to this part of themselves by building swords and guns out of various materials.

Reading Carlsson-Paige's book was a relief because I had not known what to do with my first son's need to express what seemed like aggression. Now I realize how essential a sword and shield are for protecting yourself and your energetic space. This masculine protection is the key to having good boundaries, standing up for yourself, saying no to toxicity, and cultivating a safe place for the feminine in boys or girls. Throughout our house, there are swords carved from wood and shields made from cardboard and metal, and the layers of expression that come through these masculine forms is exquisite. Boys also have a tremendous need to hit, wrestle, and throw and to externalize their energy. Learning how to manage their masculine essence is an important skill for boys, and they discover how to do this by working through its expression with other boys, in sports and other physical modes.

When my sons were three and four, their frustrations could easily turn to a spontaneous striking out. I might say, "It looks like you are feeling angry or frustrated and you have some hitting energy. You can hit a pillow or we can go outside and you can hit the ground with a stick." Another option is to redirect the hitting by throwing a ball. However, boys need to release this energy expression. Telling them to stop hitting will simply add to their frustration. Likewise, when their external energy is becoming too big for the living room, I invite them to go outside and play or to find a calm center. Or I join in the fray for a bit of roughhousing or wrestling, because the way to cultivate joyful boys is to tap into their physical fun.

Celebrate Their Beauty

There is a cultural tendency to overemphasize the appearance of girls, but the counter to that is we rarely tell our boys they are beautiful. "Gorgeous" and "beautiful" are two words my boys hear in regard to themselves several times a week. "I loved seeing you jump over that puddle; you were strong and beautiful." "When you were playing your guitar, you were radiant." "Your eyes are so clear and gorgeous."

The beauty of boys—their vitality as they streak like a shaft of light through any given moment—is hard to miss. But the *beauty* of boys—the quiet shimmer that is present in their bodies, a mostly wordless expression that is both energizing and deeply intuitive if acknowledged, is easily missed (or dismissed), which is perhaps a wound that many men carry.

I also teach my boys to honor the female body and the feminine by how I honor myself and my body. I speak of the energy opening that occurs each month with menstruation (and in a major way with birth) and allows women to "envision" and "see" for their families. I talk about the sacred blood of my bleeding time and how it nourished each one of us in the womb, as well as how its release assists me in clearing all that I hold as a woman. Boys will better know their own beauty if they understand the sacredness they came from; they will cherish the feminine and the true beauty of the future women in their lives.

In my own feminine presence, this realm of the right brain/holistic/intuitive, I see my sons and I understand the code they are working with. I want them to be aware of their own feminine creative energy that will ultimately expand the potential of their masculine forms. I admire the swords, shields, and other creations that arise, and I encourage them to continue giving full expression to their beauty. And in response, my sons, each one of them, shine.

How do you access the feminine and masculine aspects in mothering and daily life?

How can you expand these energies for yourself and your children?

What are you learning about gender, gender codes, and other ways of being?

Enhancing Positive Energy

Developing positive structures and healthy family dynamics in a house with children requires ongoing commitment and focus. With my own children, I have learned to emphasize certain energy patterns and redirect them to these optimal places. I read parenting books to enhance my overall skills with children, but I rely most on my sense of their energy to guide my response. Sometimes the response is sharp, with clear expectations and boundaries; this is a more masculine mothering response. Other times I am softer and more focused on meeting one of their needs, bringing out my feminine nature to engage what they are showing me. The main objective is to maintain equilibrium in the energy of the child and the family.

Animals can provide clues about energy and facilitating balanced energy fields. To understand energy dynamics in a household, I recommend reading any book by Cesar Millan, who is also known as the dog whisperer. He emphasizes the importance of establishing a balanced and calm energy in order to train a dog, as well as to foster a stable and balanced personality in the dog. Millan suggests cultivating a calm authority, which carries a presence that the dog will respect and respond to. It is the same with children.

Learn how to create harmony in your own energy and then use your balanced center to help you establish harmony with your children. Millan employs older, well-balanced dogs in working with puppies or dogs with unstable energy to assist their ability to live in a balanced state. To be able to cultivate balanced energy in your home, you need to find and maintain it for yourself as a mother.

When you move from a calm and balanced center, your guiding touch is more powerful than punishment in moving your child toward a desired outcome. Balancing your own center can be a simple process with the Pelvic Bowl Sings exercise (page 248). This exercise can be done regularly to establish a routine pattern of equilibrium or utilized to restore your mothering center whenever you feel out of balance.

The Importance of Establishing Boundaries

In this parenting era, there is an emphasis on connection and communication that takes into account a child's needs and forges powerful bonds. However, in this engaged process, children may feel more entitled to negotiate with their parents. Children need boundaries—the implied agreements that establish clear structure and expectations—and parents who can enforce them.

In addition to being respectful and able to get along with people, children who learn to work with boundaries have a better container for their own energy. Without boundaries, children will assume it is normal to overstep the boundaries of others. If this does not cause conflict in the home, then it will cause conflict with future teachers, employers, friends, and other community members who feel disrespected. Boundaries help us stay in our rightful space and respect the needs of others.

When behavior in our home becomes disrespectful, such as using hurtful language, talking back, or not following through on agreements, my husband and I involve our children in the process of resetting the boundaries. For example, with disrespectful words or behaviors, we make a "red list" of all the disrespectful things they can recall, and we write them on our list as not allowed. We also make clear agreements for jobs and behavior, working on them together. They are more likely to enforce house rules and fulfill agreements when they are involved in making them. Reflection is also helpful: if one brother says or does something hurtful to another or is disrespectful to a parent, they are invited to go to their room and write about how they overstepped a boundary, along with their own solutions for change.

Boundaries facilitate balance in our home. If one of our boys is complaining or being overly negative, and assuming a more basic need for food or sleep has been met, they are invited to help tend the house by doing a focused task or to write a gratitude list of all the things they are thankful for. They change their energy by pondering gratitude or doing a simple task. If they are being negative to one another, they are asked to find a way to play together or to write a gratitude list of traits they admire in their sibling.

In a Montessori catalog, I found the book *Manners*, by Aliki, which has cartoon depictions of good and bad manners. The dialogue and pictures are entertaining, and the content is helpful for teaching manners. Surprisingly, my boys often chose this book off the shelf, especially at ages four and five, when they were learning about social rules and engagement. As my youngest son said when selecting this book at bedtime, "I'm trying to learn my manners."

The Power of Staying Neutral

Staying neutral and nonreactive in regard to challenges with your children will de-energize the situation instead of adding energy to a loaded system. For example, if your children are crying, whining, arguing, refusing to complete a task, or being disrespectful and you become angry yourself, then you have added input to a high-energy situation. While this is a natural response to parenting frustrations, reactive tension in your body blocks your ground connection to the earth and your heart connection to your child. If instead you are able to stay calm, breathe into your center, and move like a force of nature—that is, neutral but still strong—then you can deflate the high-intensity energy.

A counselor whose work with parents and children I admire suggested imagining an invisible piece of tape over your mouth in instances when you are about to rant to your children about their behavior. As parental frustration mounts, it is tempting to verbally flagellate your children. However, this only disrupts your bond and rarely engages children in the manner you desire, as they are likely already in a challenging place themselves. Better to talk together later when the emotional energy has been discharged for both of you. Balance instilling respect with keeping a child's spirit alive.

A friend of mine relayed a story about her two cherished horses. One was a powerful male that intimidated people, enough that they worried for my friend's safety in choosing to ride him. The other was a small mare, the mother of the fiery male. Though the mare was small and gentle, my friend said she could put the younger horse into place with one look. In this example, the mother held power not by dominion but by her presence. Being present and meeting our children with a strong, calm presence teaches them not only to behave but also, ultimately, how to hold their own energy in a balanced and thoughtful way.

What are your mothering frustrations?
How might you work toward balance in these situations?
What embodies the power of neutral for you?

Cultivating the Positive

In our family, our overall focus is to cultivate the positive by making time to play, connect, replenish, and have fun. Even chores or homework can be enjoyable when approached as opportunities to connect as a team. We also encourage each member of the family to identify their needs rather than remain stuck in a problem. For example, children are encouraged to brainstorm solutions to resolve a situation or meet their needs. Being creative for themselves is valued, and we might say, *How do you think we can make this work?*

To maintain a positive center, children need time for quiet play and inner nourishment. They require adequate rest and space from noise or electronics as well as clear breaks from their activities and hectic schedules. Make being outside a priority in order to tap into the replenishment of earth energies and fresh air. Take meals together and honor the seasons with family rituals in order to strengthen your bonds and assist children in aligning with natural rhythms.

A particularly useful book for incorporating positive guidance to instruct behavior is *Taking Charge: Caring Discipline That Works at Home and at School*, by JoAnne Nordling. This book provides examples of challenging situations that every parent will recognize, with corresponding solutions that work. Nordling also suggests that feedback be 80 percent positive to 20 percent negative, or a ratio of four positive attentions to one negative attention. In applying the four-to-one ratio to my children, I noticed how often negative behaviors are called out while positive ones are unrecognized, not only for our children but for our partners. Positive feedback does not mean empty praise but, rather, descriptive words that show you are paying attention to what your child is doing. For example, "I noticed how you were throwing the ball with your brother and listening carefully to him. I like the way you set up a creative game together." You increase what you pay attention to. Emphasizing the positive within the family will increase the positive energy for everyone.

Nordling emphasizes the power of paying attention to a child during neutral times, when a child is simply playing quietly. In this case, you pay attention with your quiet presence, a touch, or a nod. This positive attention during neutral times conveys a sense of unconditional love to the child; it shows that they are valued for who they are rather than what they do or how they behave. When a child feels secure in your love, particularly through how you connect with and relate to them on a routine basis, they are also more likely to be in a positive frame of mind themselves.

There are many ways to cultivate the positive: moving from a place of frustration to the infinite potential of solutions, shifting a closed heart to an open one, working with energy blocks to restore flow, and transforming disequilibrium to alignment in energy balance. One of the most positive things you can do for yourself as a mother is to release all mothering guilt or regret. There are times you will not meet your children's needs or will even be hurtful toward your children, but your children are resilient and will recover. There are conflicts that will arise and events that cause pain. Address your areas of deficit as a mother or any situations that have inflicted a wound for your child, but do so with compassion rather than guilt or regret. Guilt closes down your heart center and restricts the spirit energies that will come to your assistance in the presence of self-love. Regret keeps your energy in the past, with the challenge or wound, instead of in the present where the healing can occur.

Do your mothering practice while loving yourself and recognizing the imperfection of life and relationships. Not only will you enhance your skills, but you will also teach your children how to learn and grow in a model of compassion. Saying "I'm sorry" can be a positive action. Being able to say it ourselves, to our children or partner, not only facilitates the positive but also models life skills for making harmonious relationships and recovering from conflict. As my youngest said when he was planning to apologize to his brother, "My heart wants to say sorry, but my head doesn't." Being able to express regret and access compassion requires the sometimes uncomfortable shift from head to heart, but it feels so much better once the heart is leading the way.

In witnessing our children, we see ourselves illuminated, including the places we lost touch with when we were children. As we love and tend our children, the wounded aspects of our heart can be revealed and tended to as well. The very process of mothering can heal the mothering heart.

NINE

Tending the Heart
of the Family

The next day was the summer solstice; it was my baby's due date and my husband's birthday. My first son was born on his due date, and it seemed unlikely that my third child would be born on a due date, too. Figuring I had some time before this baby arrived, I decided to take my boys to a local performance-art installation. I was intrigued by the show's description: a series of old-fashioned typewriters on which you were invited to type a love note that would be delivered by bicycle anywhere in the city. It seemed the perfect outing for my very pregnant self and my two boys, who had just wrapped up school for the summer.

We parked downtown and began what felt like the longest walk of my life. The sun beat down on the sidewalk and the glare seemed to increase my already strong contractions. My boys were suddenly resistant to going anywhere, and one of them refused to walk.

Between the glaring sun, the growing contractions, my swollen belly, and my boys' resistance, I had little patience left.

In recent mornings, I had awakened with contractions strong enough to make me wonder whether the baby's birth was imminent. Including my miscarriage, this was my fourth pregnancy and birthing experience, yet I felt as if I knew less about birth instead of more. The innocence of my first birth also meant that I was not trying to make sense of every sensation in my body like I was now. With each contraction, my mind attempted to categorize what was happening based on previous births.

I reminded myself of the spiritual path of mothering. I tried to return my mind to the openness of the beginner's mind—one that is aware of the fresh potential of the present moment, rather than focusing on accumulated knowledge that may be irrelevant. This practice of keeping an open mind is helpful as I mother my children. Otherwise I project what I think they will experience or who they will be by each behavior that arises. Keeping my focus on the present moment seemed an essential preparation for this birth event; we were planning a home birth, with all family members a part of the process, yet our plan would ultimately follow the flow of this birth and its energy.

I hoisted my youngest son onto my hip. We continued our long walk for several blocks past where I thought the installation would be. Reading about it in the newspaper, under the cool air of the ceiling fan, I had imagined an inspired adventure. Feeling the white heat rise from the city streets, stopping to breathe through each contraction, coaxing my boys toward something I was now not sure they would even enjoy, I was hoping this was not one of those times when something that seemed like a good idea fell flat.

Finally I spotted a woman with shockingly pink hair leaving a building. Bicycles were parked out front. This must be the place. I set my son down and herded both boys in her direction. We pulled open the door of an old storefront that had been converted into the art installation. The air was cool inside. Several desks sat at seemingly random places around the room. These desks each held one ancient-looking typewriter and a thick sheaf of paper. At each desk, a person hunched over the typewriter, carefully composing a love note. The love-note paper was the same shade of pink as the hair of the woman who had led us there.

Overhead, a thick rope wrapped around several bike wheels that had been converted into a series of pulleys. "Cool!" said my seven-year-old. We watched as a dark-haired young man completed his love note. He then fastened it to the thick rope with a clothespin. Another young man, standing on a platform in a bright pink jumpsuit, shouted, "Love on the line!" and began to turn a wheel that moved the rope through the pulleys. The note bounced in transit around the edge of the room.

We saw the note advancing toward a young woman dressed from head to toe in sparkles and several shades of pink. When the note arrived, she carefully removed it from the line and rolled it up. She placed it into a pale blue bottle. We watched her address the bottle before setting it into a basket full of blue-bottled notes awaiting delivery. Maybe it was the impending birth or the playful energy in the room, but a sensation of giddiness waved through my body.

A Labor of Love

We awaited our turn at a typewriter. Serious business, this love-note writing, and those composing notes took their time. Some love-note composers had focused expressions, and one had his eyes closed. I wondered what they were writing and to whom. Many of these love-note compositions required several sheets of hot-pink paper.

Sitting with my sons, surrounded by this creativity in motion, I made a silent note to nurture those early creative seeds within each of them: *May they see their own beauty and make a life from this place, rather than waiting for others to discover it.*

"Mom, there's a typewriter for us!" My son pulled me toward the table. I showed him how to press the keys to spell out a note. "Let's write a note for Daddy since it's his birthday tomorrow," I said.

My oldest typed out, "H-A-P-P-Y B-I-R-T-H-D-A-Y D-A-D-D-Y!" My four-year-old typed: "aaaaaaaaaaaaaa yyyyzyyyyyy," and then hopped off of my lap to watch a note traveling around the pulley-rope system. I added, "W-e l-o-v-e y-o-u." I touched my belly. *What do you want to say, baby?* My body responded with a strong contraction. "S-e-e y-o-u s-o-o-n! l-o-v-e, b-a-b-y," I typed, and then pulled our hot-pink note out of the typewriter, which *zinged* in response.

We pinned our note to the rope with a clothespin. Hot-pink-pantsuit guy yelled, "Love on the line!"

Away our note bounced around the edge of the room. Suddenly the rope pulley snapped apart. My boys gasped, but our note stayed clipped to the rope.

"That is some kind of love!" shouted hot-pink-pantsuit guy. "Explosive!"

"Yes, and I'm in labor," I said.

"A labor of love," sang sparkly girl.

Then in one smooth motion, pantsuit guy rescued the fallen rope, climbed a ladder, and tied the two ends together. Our note continued to bounce along to sparkly girl. Then it was rolled and placed in the basket to be delivered to our house sometime tomorrow or the next day. We floated back to our car; the kids were in the flow now, and I felt lighter, too. The giddiness stayed with me long after the boys were asleep. I wondered which would arrive first— our baby or our hot-pink love note.

Creative Collaboration: A Family Birth Event

In the waning light of the solstice eve, I sensed the potential for our baby's birth. Weeks earlier, we'd prepared our basement fire room for the birth, cleaning and blessing the space. On this night, we worked together in making the final preparations.

It felt like our own art installation as we set up the birth space: a beautiful altar, a spacious birth tub, freshly split cedar wood in the fireplace. The boys decided they would wear swimsuits when they joined me in the birth tub and ran upstairs to find them. I smiled as they placed their suits next to the empty birth tub, each one smoothing out the wrinkles.

After a long day of light, the darkness set in, and I paced the house with a restlessness. Knowing that the intensity of full labor can come at any time and require an extended and unknown amount of energy, I talked myself back into bed to rest.

Though my contractions had been intense for days, my intuition was to call the midwives in the early morning hours of the solstice. When the midwife and her assistant arrived, they checked my cervix, finding that it was about three centimeters dilated—still early labor. Then they bedded down in the room next to the birth space to see what daylight might bring.

I watched the last hours of darkness turn to early dawn light, resting in my bed, talking to my baby. As the sun's rays reached my window, I rose. As soon as I placed my feet on the floor, my water broke. This was my sign that labor was truly beginning. A feeling of anticipation flooded my body. I tiptoed out of the room so as not to awaken my sons, but my oldest son sat up out of a sound sleep, saying, "Are you in labor, Mom?"

"Yes, honey, I am," I answered.

I was about to add, "Let's be quiet so your brother can continue to sleep." But before I could speak, he leapt out of bed, saying, "Mama's in labor, baby! Rock and roll!"

His brother bolted upright and cried out, "Mama!" He reached for me. I gathered him into my arms, savoring their excitement. The golden light now filled each room. I heard my husband in the kitchen and the midwives stirring downstairs. The house was awake; the birth would begin.

We called our friends who would be the support for our boys. Both of them answered the phone and agreed to come right over. I told them there was no rush, thinking we had plenty of time. But the birth unfolded rapidly. I moved from stirring oatmeal at the stove, with strong contractions, to climbing into the just-filled birth tub with contractions that required my entire focus. We called our midwives back from the cafe on the corner, where they had gone to have breakfast in anticipation of a day of laboring. Our friends arrived. The fire was lit, the first morning birds were singing, and within twenty minutes I was in full transition.

Transition is that profound moment when the uterus has fully dilated, the birth field is aligned, and the baby moves down the vaginal canal and into the world. My energy skills had come fully to life now. I could sense that my energy body had expanded to encompass the room. The fire room ritual and retreat space, which we had made after our second son was born, felt sacred and protected. I let my energy body fill the whole space.

The Creative Energy Aligns the Flow

My oldest son was there throughout the birth, just as he had wanted to be. My second son came down the stairs to the basement as I was pushing, just as he had said he would. My husband was near my head at the edge of the birth tub. After making breakfast, filling the tub, and gathering wood for the fire, he could stay with me. Our German shepherd, Kiva, looked in at me when my husband carried wood through the basement door that connected to our yard. She was the guardian of both our family and the energy of our home. I rested, knowing she would be on watch.

The birth was intense in the final moments. The birth energy surged through me, calling to mind a wild horse. I was thankful for the water cushioning my pelvis. I placed my hand at my perineum and guided my midwife's hand there as well. I wanted to support my stretching tissues and also keep my focus on this root entry point. The ripples of birth moving through me kept expanding my energy outward. I knew that I needed to maintain my focus on the root to bring our baby down and out.

In each of my births, and my miscarriage, there had been a pause right before the entry. I imagine this is preparation for the first crossing over through the spirit door. Just as before, I felt the pause in my center. I could not have spoken any words at this point, but inside myself I said to my baby, *I'm ready to meet you.*

With these words, he was born. I felt the release of his body coming from mine. I reached down into the water to lift him to my chest. My sense of self had expanded beyond my body and my arms. The midwives wrapped a towel across my chest to cover his body and keep him warm. My sons, in their swimsuits, climbed into the tub with us. The baby's dark eyes opened slightly to take in this family gathered around him. We would have the day to savor him. It was just eight thirty in the morning on the longest day of the year.

A few hours after my son was born, I heard the distinct sound of a bicycle bell. I was resting in bed with the new baby. The messenger saw my husband in our side yard and handed him a bottle with the love note we had written the day before. Our hot-pink love note was a surprise, delivered on his birthday—and now the birthday of one of his sons. My husband came to me with the crisp note in his hand; the creative energy had aligned, with our baby's birth and love-note delivery as one fluid orchestration.

Having a Creative Practice with Children

Women often ask me how I was able to write my first book while birthing and then mothering three children. The key lies within the previous story: allowing the creative flow from my center to guide me as both a mother and creative being. Honing my ability to follow this flow, with a few specific techniques, enables my practice as a healer and writer and makes mothering its own creative process. I incorporate these principles for daily inspiration in order to bring my creative essence into all aspects of my life. The transformative process of becoming a mother is the ultimate creative inspiration; your life, your motherpiece, is the art.

Engaging Your Creative Essence

I engage my inner creative self in the *process* of creating rather than focusing on a particular outcome or product. I follow the creative flow arising from my family's rhythm and my own center. For example, today is a warm spring Sunday, inviting us outside to explore. But my youngest son awoke with a fever. Most people would not see this as a creative moment, but with the open timing that sickness brings as regular activities fall away, I engage my creative energy. With his illness and need for rest, the creative flow turns inward. I shift my focus to match his needs. Many of the chapters of my previous book were written during nap times with young children or while tending to one who was ill, sometimes writing even while they were resting in my lap.

Creativity is more about engaging an energy and the essence of life than it is about creating something specific. Writing engages my own creative flow in such a way that a vibrant energy surrounds us. This creative spark brings a comfort, lightness, and support for my own needs during an inward time that otherwise might feel isolating. When I access my creative potential, I also notice that my children often respond by being more creative themselves or, if they are not feeling well, by settling into a deep peace. Today my son needs my presence, and we may barely leave the bedroom. But we will both feel the rejuvenation that comes from engaging the creative field.

Now I can hear that my older son, who is downstairs, has picked up his ukulele and is playing music. I have found that no matter where they are in the house, if I step into my creative space, my sons feel this change in the energy. They begin to engage their own creative essence in making music, drawing, or building elaborate Lego spaceships. I am following the invitation to create, and so are they.

Committing to Your Creative Craft

Every woman can feel more creative if she picks one or two creative pursuits that are her first priority. Rather than clean or do the dishes when an opening presents itself, my first movement is to write. This is like growing a garden. Weeding or mulching a small amount with each opportunity to tend the field makes a bountiful garden over time.

This commitment means prioritizing your needs as a creative being and giving yourself permission to be creative even while mothering. It may require letting go of expectations for a perfectly organized house or not finishing tasks in order to focus on your creative process. Many mothers I have worked with feel guilty when they do something for themselves. Ironically, you have much more to give when you cultivate your own creativity. Accessing your creative essence on a regular basis enriches your energy and the energy you bring to your children. If you are happy and fulfilled, your children will sense and draw from this capacity.

Showing your children that you are a creative being with unique attributes gives them permission to tap into their own creative essence. Encourage them to find their own creative passions. Creative expression is the best resource for making a vibrant life. Knowing their own creative potential will come in handy for solving problems, finding life-giving partnerships, directing their life force, making a career, and setting up healthy practices for living.

When my first son was about nine, he began to worry about what he was "going to do for a living." Perhaps they had been talking about careers at school. Redirecting him to his center, I assured him that his creative essence would guide his path. The creative essence within is a powerful force for creating our lives. When we tune in to our creative potential while mothering, we not only make a meaningful life for ourselves but we also model for our children how to make one for themselves.

Forging a Feminine-Masculine Model

Living in alignment with a feminine-masculine model means learning how to alternate between the dreamy feminine state of creative inspiration and the masculine realm of outward expression and form. If you only access the feminine, you feel constantly inspired but never finish a visible creation. Or you may feel creative but forget to tend to the basics of living, like cleaning your house, paying the bills, or making a meal. If you only access the masculine, you are constantly crossing items off your to-do list but feel generally tired or uninspired. To have a creative life that both nourishes you and gives you something to show for your efforts, you need to access both the feminine and masculine aspects of your creative range.

In my life, when the muse strikes, I write down the inspiration I have received and I put the piece of paper into a folder. It may be a workshop idea, a topic for one of my classes, a way to engage with my children, or a theme for an article or book. The information comes in a flash, when I wake up, take a shower, or even in the midst of my day, but there is usually not time in that moment to express it fully. So I make a quick note and tuck it into a file, giving my feminine inspiration a place to land.

Later, when the opportunity arises or I have a set work time on my schedule, I then expand the workshop idea or piece of writing. Taking time to craft a writing project is my masculine aspect, giving form to my creative energy and being specific in my doing. The feminine and masculine are very different aspects and even represent two dimensions of the creative field. The feminine is more fluid and expansive, bringing in the raw energy of inspiration. The masculine is more focused and task-oriented, to direct and give shape to the energy. Working with both aspects will make the best creative products and expressions. The feminine invites a creative flow, and the masculine directs the flow into a tangible form.

Having a creative practice in making art, gardening, knitting, cooking, or whatever you enjoy gives you a hands-on connection to the beauty within, which restores your deepest wells. Your creative practice is the secret to cultivating a creative life and bountiful motherhood. Hold space for this creative practice by making it a priority and access its energy by following the rhythms that arise in each season of mothering.

Manifesting Your Creative Dreams

Every woman benefits by accessing the creative potential in her center and cultivating it with intention. Birthing a child stimulates this creative essence within, but this essence can be accessed on a daily basis to create a woman's dreams—whether in the form of a partnership, a family, a way of life, a career, or a work of art. Tapping into this flow can enhance the creative aspects of mothering, bring in more nourishment, assist the balance between outer work and inner home life, or reestablish the connection to a creative pursuit. The creative essence within each one of us is related to our soul purpose and contains immeasurable value in our lives.

One key to being able to create your dreams is to establish both a short-term and long-term orientation. Make a long-term creative plan but maintain your focus on the short-term tasks that align with your plan. First formulate a creative road map for yourself: write down five to seven long-term intentions. Then work incrementally each day toward a particular creative intention: draw, meditate, try a new recipe, take your kids to a wild place, join a class, explore a new professional field, wear a different style or color for yourself. Long-term focus sets the tone for your overall creative essence, but the expression of this essence comes by letting each day guide and inspire the direction of your creative flow.

Mike Dooley, author of *Manifesting Change*, suggests envisioning what the "big picture," or end point, of your creative dreams looks like. This means that rather than thinking through how to manifest your creative desires, you imagine how it feels when they are fully realized. In this way, you energize their potential. Then take a step or two each day in the direction of your creative visions.

Doing a small task with routine focus will build your energy in a sustainable manner. If you are becoming overwhelmed or feeling creatively frustrated, you are very likely taking on too much at once or expecting major results without investing in regular short-term sessions over an extended period. Keep your creative attention in the present moment of creative flow and, with patience and careful tending, you will achieve long-term objectives.

Exercise: Setting Your Creative Intentions

1. Take a moment to connect to your creative center and reflect on this capacity within. Receive what is here for you.

2. After centering yourself, call to mind your top five to seven creative goals for the next year. Write them on a piece of paper.

3. Now make a vision for each of these goals in their fully realized form, just like an athlete visualizes his or her full potential before taking action.

4. When you have finished visualizing each creative goal, look at your written list to see if they need any modification. Notice which ones are a priority right now.

5. Find a place for this list. Once a week, read it over and visualize these creative intentions. If you find that your creative energy is regularly aligned with your intentions, celebrate this achievement. If not, recalibrate your focus as needed. Let spirit guide your way for bringing these intentions into reality with synchronicities, opportunities, and the flow of daily life.

6. After one year, set new intentions to continue navigating toward your creative dreams.

Be Inspired—Do What You Love

We talk about "doing what you love" in regard to a career. It also applies directly to mothering from the center and activating your creativity. Do what you love and bring it into the center of your family life. For me, this means giving and receiving bodywork, incorporating family ritual, inviting an awareness and relationship with spirit, going to wild places, and making space for creative flow in writing, walking, or daydreaming. By involving your children in the activities you love, you raise the joy for you and your family; this is wild mothering.

Savor the unexpected bliss and unformed potential of your nonlinear days with your children. Receive the unexpected blessings (like when, on day three of sleeplessly tending my young son through an illness, he threw his arms around my neck, saying, "I sure do love you, Mama"). Create family fun by taking walks, having treats, playing games, reading books, planning vacations, or making a day outing to nature. Follow your children's lead toward play. Put on music and dance or sing together. Exchange back massages. Watch a movie. Cook together on a cold day or make a fire. Set down work or uninspiring tasks and do something that feels good until you are rejuvenated. Stretch, sit in the sun, hang out with your kids, just be. At the end of your day, reflect on what caught your attention or was good for your soul to reinforce your ability to notice the simple daily inspirations.

Cultivating Happiness: Engaging the Energy

How do you find happiness? Kids, like most people, tend to find happiness not through heightened stimulation or vast leisure but by engaging their energy. My challenge as a mother is to remain neutral through the demands or complaints of boredom, gently making suggestions until my children find their own way—which they eventually do—sometimes entering their most creative part of the day. I want them to realize that being happy can be a relatively simple task and that it is within their power to create their own happiness.

Dr. Tal Ben-Shahar researches the creation and maintenance of happiness. As the father of two children, he also relates his findings to parenting. In his book *Happier*, Ben-Shahar discusses the idea that while happiness is thought of as having the freedom to be idle and indulge in our pleasures, most people are actually happier by participating in an activity.

In the summer months, when leisure is more prominent in my family's life, I find this to be true. While my children fantasize about having "nothing to do" in the summer, they are also more prone to conflict and frustration (and so am I) when we have no schedule to organize our energy around. It takes several weeks to switch into summer mode, but as my children (and our family) find a more organic rhythm to structure our days, we also become happier.

Teaching Kids to Cultivate Their Own Happiness

In previous generations, parents rarely considered whether or not their children were happy. As a result, emotional needs largely were internalized or went unaddressed. Now, however, children's emotional needs are continuously monitored, and parents may be overly concerned with their children's happiness.

To compensate for the emotional deficits that they experienced, many parents of this generation have gone to great lengths to address the emotional needs of their children. Attending to emotional well-being can be more straightforward with toddlers. Much of the time, they are satisfied by ample hugs, playtime, rest, and snacks. As children grow, how to best address their emotional needs becomes significantly more complicated.

Educators are talking about an increasing sense of entitlement in young people. My husband and I have given our children a voice and ability to make choices in many aspects of their lives. We seek to empower them and foster a robust emotional nature. Yet these frequent choices can also result in expectations that they can negotiate everything. When I say no to a new book, toy, item of candy, a later bedtime, and so on, suddenly one of them is challenging my answer with a plethora of negotiation tactics. I wonder how this will affect their ability to work hard or accept challenges later on. In fact, several psychologists are writing about the trend in young people to be increasingly unhappy because they have developed little tolerance for stress or discomfort.

Worrying about our children's happiness in every interaction or being too connected to their emotional nature can cause us to interfere with their own ability to self-regulate. I have had an extended nursing relationship with my children. I have co-slept and carried them with me through all their early years. Our connection is so close that I can feel their crush of disappointment as if it were my own. The caretaker in me wants to fix the situation or make it better, but I see how doing so is a disservice to them in the long run.

Instead, I make it a practice to stay in connection with them but detach from the emotions they are feeling, as if I am an observer to the situation. In this way, I offer support with my presence and encouragement to work it out for themselves. Trusting their ability to handle emotional discomfort allows them to trust themselves as well. Each little challenge or pain they encounter ultimately prepares them for the ebb and flow of life.

Childhood boredom is another place for developing emotional resilience. Often, outside the structure of school hours or activities, one of my children will announce that he is bored. On impulse, I want to sweep them off to an adventure and take away that boredom. I imagine us going to the water park or rock-climbing gym. I have, in fact, tried to chase away boredom with an exciting activity, only to learn that it often does not work anyway. Either the activity is a disappointment or the boredom returns as soon as the fun is over, and then I am frustrated that they are not more appreciative. This is when I have to remember that making my kids happy is not the ultimate goal; my goal is to teach them to cultivate their own happiness.

Being Known Rather Than Validated

According to Ben-Shahar, another key for happiness is being known as a unique individual, rather than simply validated. Of the women I see in my practice, one of their greatest desires is to be known for their authentic selves and seen for their inherent beauty. Perhaps one essential ingredient in family happiness is that each member feels known within the group.

As mothers, we can know our children better if we know ourselves. By tuning in to our own center and core essence, we have the presence from which to witness the radiance of our children and even our partner. From this knowing comes an attunement with life and an aliveness that we can cultivate and share as a family.

Likewise, it is essential that we know our needs as mothers and as creative women. Mothering and all the demands that arise in the process of tending children and the home or balancing work and home can be immensely challenging. Certainly there are moments of brilliant and unexpected joy in the presence of children. But finding joy—or enjoyment—as a routine set point is a true practice that requires knowing how to deal with stress, having good structures of support, and making space for what truly makes you happy.

Accessing Spontaneous Joy

Happiness is a way of being that can be tapped into at any moment by calling your attention to the present. The other day when I was working at home, my older sons were entertaining themselves and my youngest son played with a babysitter. After spending the morning playing together, my older sons began to argue intensely. Instead of encouraging them to work it out, which needs to happen when I have a particular work deadline, I invited them to take a walk with me in the warmth of the gentle August day.

We walked and talked about whatever came through our minds, my older son gliding along on his new cruiser skateboard and my other son holding my hand. I asked if I could try riding the board. I stepped onto the smooth koa wood as my sons held me protectively from each side. With their arms around me, I rolled along through the sweet air, savoring the beauty of being with these boys.

Exercise: Energizing the Moment

1. Notice what is happening in this moment. How are you feeling? Where are you? Is there a sense of peace around you, or

is something in need of tending? If you are with your children, how are they? What are they doing presently?

2. Focus on the beauty you can access right now. Set down any work and simply breathe. Look outside to see what is happening in the sky. Sense the expansiveness around you.

3. Reflect on your loves and places of gratitude. Energize the space around you with the blessings of your life. Sense how this changes the energy.

4. Now engage the moment with intention. See your children; notice their eyes and the expression on their faces. Join their play with your full presence. Give a family member a heartfelt touch or embrace. Turn on music and have a dance party with your children. Reach out and call a friend. Simply savor this energy potential.

5. Step back into your previous task or redirect yourself; carry the energy of this blessed moment with you through your day. Try bringing this energized presence to a mothering task, like bathing your child or tending the house, and see what changes.

The Power of Energetic Resonance

Resonance in sound is defined as a quality of depth, fullness, and reverberation. When a sound achieves resonance, it has a balanced and pleasing tonal pattern. I further define resonance energetically, as a way of aligning ourselves to create a vibration of harmony rather than discord. Harmony in sound patterns creates music, while harmony in the energy field makes beauty as well. Learning to cultivate your own harmonic resonance is a powerful tool for influencing or aligning with an energy potential. It facilitates a harmonious resonance in the home and with your children.

To cultivate a harmonic resonance, it helps to know what brings a sense of harmony to your own being. For me, taking deep breaths calms my center. Seeing my children—not simply seeing what they are doing but actually touching them or looking into their eyes—brings more resonance between us. It is also helpful to move my body so that the energy flows more readily. Stepping outside and observing the seasonal changes in my yard brings resonance with the earth's energy. Going to a wild place naturally cultivates resonance. Blessings create a resonance with the divine: *May we be blessed. May we be held. Thank you for the blessing of this moment. Please guide us. May we receive our inspiration.*

Developing Your Resonance

Resonance is a pattern of alignment, a way of harmonizing in a synchronous vibration. In my women's health practice, I teach women to find the resonance between the center of their bodies, the earth's energy, and the divine creative essence that fuels life. Too often, as women developing careers, we have learned to find resonance with our professions and work lives. These external demands have little to do with our own health, well-being, or the more internal realms of spirit, the hearth of the home, and raising children. Or we internalize patterns of stress rather than resonance. As a mother, developing resonance with your inner creative capacity is essential for accessing your creative resources and for navigating the demands and stress of caretaking in a manner that replenishes rather than depletes your energy field.

One of my favorite exercises for creating resonance in the center is a brief four-minute meditation called Pelvic Bowl Sings, which I do whenever I want to align the energy in my bowl. Imagine a singing bowl and the harmonic vibration that radiates out from the center as the singing bowl finds its frequency. When a singing bowl is played, the harmonic vibration invites those listening to attune in a synchronous manner. If you have ever listened to a singing bowl or even a piece of music that moves you, you often find yourself becoming more relaxed and open, even inspired. In this way, energy is exchanged when two systems—in this case, a form of music and a person—come into alignment at a certain frequency.

Exercise: Pelvic Bowl Sings

1. *Center.* Whatever you are doing now, find your center. Drop down to this internal creative place within yourself. Take note of how you are feeling in this space. Sense the present state of your creative and mothering energy. Remember, you can choose the quality of the energy you hold in your center.

2. *Clear.* Clarify your bowl by sweeping the energy with your inner awareness. Walk around your pelvic bowl and sweep as you go. Give permission for your body to clear anything that no longer serves you. On each inhale of your breath, imagine fresh energy rejuvenating your center. With each exhale, invite a full release.

3. *Balance.* Balance the inner fire (feminine) and the outer fire (masculine) to move your creative flow in a dynamic and sustainable manner. Focus on your left ovary and send breath to this feminine fire. Invite your feminine radiance to nourish and inspire your center. Now focus on your right ovary and send breath to this masculine fire. Invite your masculine radiance to give full expression to your creative essence. Mothering can be a creative practice when you align these core fires.

4. *Bless.* In your womb space, the sacred altar for receiving divine energy, set your top creative intentions. Connect your heart and womb; let the love flow through your center. Call on the sacred to bless your intentions and to assist your mothering. Invite the brilliance of spirit to fill your bowl. Relish this shimmering light; remember that you are sacred. Embody your radiance.

5. *Sing.* Walk around your pelvic bowl and celebrate this space. Feel the resonance arise as you cherish your center. Take this resonance and engage your full capacity to live and mother with creative expression. Meeting each ordinary or extraordinary moment from your center, your pelvic bowl sings.

Creating Family Resonance

If you are holding a harmonic pattern in your center, you will influence your family to resonate with you. The stronger your ability to hold this frequency, the easier it is to maintain it in times of stress, such as conflict with your partner, a child's tantrum, or even a visit with your family of origin. When it is difficult to hold your own centered frequency, a child's tantrum or other challenge can pull you from your center and influence your resonance. In this case, you may become stressed and amplify the stress frequency.

Finding a place of centered resonance—especially in the presence of stress—is how we enhance understanding, trust, connection, and love with one another. Learning to establish centered resonance with your child, your partner, or your family is one of the most powerful energy tools for cultivating harmony in your home. Playing a game or simply tossing a football can create a family resonance.

Animals play a role in resonance as well. A calm and centered animal companion can bring a greater resonance of connection and positive energy flow, just as one who is not having his or her needs met can add to the chaos. The healing effect of animals, and their ability to bring people into a resonant state, is the basis for pet therapy. Our family has long been tended by our German shepherd, Kiva, who protects and watches over our family energy field. We also have two parrots that reflect the state of our family field—biting or squawking when there are disruptions in the field and people are cranky, or chirping, fluffing their feathers, and rubbing their heads against our hands when there is ease and the heart energy is flowing strongly.

Children and whole families often align themselves with the energy of the mother. *If mama ain't happy, ain't nobody happy.* Knowing how to generate a positive resonance as a woman and a mother, by practicing presence and energy alignment in your own field, is a potent resource for maintaining the family resonance.

Attuning to Energetically Sensitive Children
Some children are particularly sensitive to energy or changes in energy. Understanding resonance can be helpful in working with these children. Sensitive children are noticeably affected by making transitions, going outside the home or spending time with others (particularly in high-intensity situations). They may be more likely to have a tantrum, be highly expressive regarding their sense of discomfort, or otherwise express their sensitivity.

For energetically sensitive children and babies, bodywork is calming and can help them better process energy and other sensory information. As a parent, using touch—and fewer words—can assist a child's ability to "hear" and respond. When working with the energy connection to your sensitive child, tuning within and sensing the connection, rather than reacting to a particular challenge, is also highly beneficial.

Energy-sensitive children are adept at both sensing and picking up on energy. If they are having a difficult day, it is time to clear the energy field of the home. Frequently it is the energy, not the child, that is the problem. With focus on clarifying the energy field, the child typically becomes calm. Prepare a spiritual bath (page 13) and bless your home and each family member. These children can alert us to subtle imbalances in the energy field long before others sense them. Empower your child to know that they are sensitive, and teach them how to clear their own field as well as to be aware of changes in energy. The ability to sense energy can be a tremendous gift when energy practices are incorporated in parenting these highly attuned children.

Resonance as a Practice

Finding and maintaining a pattern of energetic harmony or resonance in your center can radically shift how you embody your world. Many of us have learned or inherited patterns of overworking ourselves, internalizing stress, or feeling a generalized scarcity, and these patterns become our default way of being. Resonance as a practice allows you to change the inherited patterns of how you access and use your creative energy. For example, if anger was the strongest or most frequent energy current in your family of origin, practicing a new pattern of resonance that instead energizes your love and blessings will change the way you live and experience your life.

Resonance as a practice means cultivating a core harmony that energizes your center, regardless of the circumstances or outer events of your life. Resonance even guides you toward joy and self-care. Rather than feeling good or balanced only when things are happening well, you have this positive feeling or resonance pattern with you at all times that can add to your enjoyment of a particular moment and assist you with any challenges. Instead of static patterns, which set you up for rigid responses to life or parenting, resonance puts you in touch with the dynamic and infinitely creative potential within.

Maintaining harmony while mothering is ideal for honing your resonance skills because children are inherently spontaneous and unpredictable. Apply resonance to counter the stress of parenting or to find a peaceful center when a child is in the midst of an emotional storm. Especially after a day of school, children may be more emotionally charged because each one of them is navigating hundreds of social encounters and the pressures of assignments, and they are learning to process the stress, stimuli, joys, and challenges of engaging in the world. Emotional meltdowns or discharges are a normal part of letting off steam, although they are not an excuse for being disrespectful. Cultivating your own inner harmonic resonance not only helps you in encountering these challenges with your children, but it also invites them to be present with what is happening, to have skills for restoring resonance with a peaceful state in themselves, and to be accountable for their own energy.

Developing centered resonance in daily mothering helps you show true unconditional love to your children, which translates as *I can see and connect with you even when you are having a hard time. In fact, when you are having a hard time, I know that you need our connection most of all.* Isn't that what we all want? Resonance skills not only assist connection with children, but they also improve our ability to be compassionate with ourselves and our partner. Practicing resonance with my husband, I see more clearly his weariness or my own weariness and our need for tangible expressions of love. This practice enhances our ability to find resonance together, even during the challenging moments, of which parenting offers many.

This brings us to the most important point: the more we have presence in our centers and resonance with the type of energy we want to hold there, the more we will meet and thus teach our families to live from this place as well. We have the power to choose what energy we hold in the center. Instead of being overwhelmed by a to-do list, you may notice the blossoms outside your window. Rather than focusing on a place of stress with a child or partner, you can identify needs and think creatively about solutions. By attuning with the simple joys of mothering, your energy will flow more readily and allow you to counter any difficulties. Finding resonance in ourselves and with one another is essential for sharing our love and receiving the gifts of a life made together.

Women's Stories: Engaging Her Creative Resonance

One of my clients, Gina, came for pelvic work one day. When she entered my office, she was visibly frustrated. Gina had had a stressful morning with her husband and two children and felt that leaving the house for her own self-care had been a monumental task. I concurred with her that mothering can be immensely challenging, sometimes for days or weeks in a row. But I also invited her to tune in to her own energy pattern, which was amplifying rather than dissipating the stress.

We began with a meditation to establish resonance in her pelvic bowl. With direct focus on her own body, Gina recognized the tension pattern in her core. She was clenching her pelvic muscles and breathing in a shallow manner, as if guarding against the stress. However, holding tension in the body reduces energy flow. The effects of stress and feelings of pressure escalate as a result of this holding pattern.

I invited Gina to acknowledge the pattern in her center and to pay attention to the specific sensations it caused. She felt pressure, as if things were closing in on her, particularly in her lower belly. Her energy had a sinking sensation, as if it were draining from her body like water from a bathtub. In noticing these sensations, Gina realized that she felt responsible for the happiness of everyone in her family. She felt as if she were failing at her mothering unless they were all happy. Receiving this information, she also realized that this definition of happiness meant that no one had any emotions that seemed *negative*, like sadness, frustration, anger, and so on. This was an unconscious desire on her part, and she recognized how frantically she tended the emotional state of the family to avoid any expression that might overwhelm her.

When we unravel the deeper emotional patterns we carry, they are often reaction patterns from our own childhood. In Gina's case, there had been a high level of conflict and stress between her parents. They fought with aggression and lashed out at Gina and her siblings, so that emotional energy carried a psychic weight instead of being a normal part of expression.

I encouraged Gina to acknowledge this pattern and then release it from her core energy field. In part, feeling responsible for others' feelings is also an unconscious attempt to control the emotional energies and maintain a "safe" range. Clearing the energetic stress around emotional expression will release the need to control the emotional energies. Gina breathed from her center and down into the earth, giving her body permission to release what no longer served her. In working with the energy, I suggest sensing the energy release or using the inner eye to see it move from the body. It is helpful to both sense and visualize energy in order to engage the energy field around the body and facilitate resonance.

Gina's pelvis became hot as the energy cleared. She also released responsibility for holding the emotional energy for the family. While mothers tune in to the emotional energy of their family members and assist the flow, they do not have the capacity to carry these extra energies. Gina's center cooled as the energy burden diminished. I asked Gina to imagine a vision of her family in their most vibrant form. She saw an image of them at an ocean beach, playing alongside the incoming waves. Imagining a place in nature is helpful for realizing that there are greater energies to hold the family. The earth energy and the Great Mother essence can hold them; mothers can call upon these greater energies to assist the nurturing of family flow.

Gina focused on three intentions to support her family vision: to make her creative resonance a priority; to take her family to the ocean and on other adventures on a regular basis; and to invite each family member to actively participate in cultivating family harmony. As she set these intentions in her center, she noticed the difference in herself. Her pelvis had released the tension and now felt dynamically engaged. Instead of being stuck and overwhelmed, her center pulsed with potential. Gina left my office with her new resonant form and, like a singing bowl, invited her family to attune there as well.

Mother as Visionary

Mothers have the potential to sense the family energy, which is why they are sensitive to any stress or energy imbalances. They can also more clearly see or sense the needs of their children or family, which is a gift but may at times feel burdensome. How many mothers have said to their partner, "Why can't you see what I do?"

Rather than taking responsibility for the energy of those in her family, a mother does well to recognize her innate ability and access this potential for visualizing the overall family energy field and flow. It is like steering a ship rather than tending to each of the shipmates individually; if a mother focuses on the direction of the family flow, then she can steer the energy in beneficial ways. She can envision the capacity of a child and guide the activities to develop their creative expression and life skills.

As my first son turned eight, I saw the first glimpses of him beyond childhood. I realized that his father's masculine essence (as well as modeling from other males) was essential for him in becoming a man. Yet my son expressed his masculine energy primarily in playing sports. His father was athletic but did not have an affinity for playing team sports. I wondered how they would engage their male aspects with one another, particularly since men are no longer hunting for the tribe and spending vast periods of time in nature together. I could not solve this dilemma directly, so I called them to mind in my capacity as family visionary.

I thought about my husband's male expression. It was primarily through music and activities like mountain biking and running. A guitar class came to mind; perhaps they could take a guitar class together. I made the suggestion to my husband for a father-son guitar class, and, after finding a teacher, they began their joint venture. Now, after many guitar classes, musical equipment purchases, and concerts, they have created a rich expression of male connection (along with mountain biking, stand-up paddling, and becoming fans of the local professional soccer team). Of course, my husband remembers the guitar class as his idea.

Whenever there is an imbalance or a challenge in the family flow, mothers can envision potential ways to realign the energy or tend connections. Likewise, organizing the family structure for replenishment, vacations, wellness, and play is more easily done by the person in the center of the flow. This can feel like additional work but only if a mother is taking everything on as her responsibility. If she engages her creative energy to perceive and align the overall family flow, then it is her power.

Exercise: Making a Family Vision

1. Imagine your family in its most vibrant and resonant form. Let the vision become clear. This is your family potential.

2. What are you doing together in this vision? Where are you? Sense the way you feel. Notice the energy. Listen.

3. Is everyone in your family present in your vision? Are there any places that need more tending or relationships between members that need support for more vibrance? What energy can you intentionally cultivate as a family?

4. Set three intentions to create or support this family vision. What will bring this family resonance into your days together? How can it assist any challenges?

5. Give thanks for the blessing of your family. Thank each member for the gifts and beauty they bring.

6. Give thanks for yourself as mother. Set an intention for your own creative expression. Let radiant energy surround you and replenish you on all levels. Recognize yourself as a blessing, and receive blessing energy into your center.

7. Carry this resonance into your mothering; let your vision come to life. In day to day reality, remember the potential.

A Sacred Passage

As the family visionary, I both see and align the flow for our family rhythm. Just as with the births of each of my children, I sensed a profound energy in this particular day ahead of me. It was another warm August day, like the day of my miscarriage many years before. I awoke early as the sun rose and went out to our backyard where Kiva, our fourteen-year-old German shepherd, lay, unable to get up. Coming before any of our children, she had tended and protected the heart of our family. In a house full of males, she was my co-mother. On her last day with us, I bore witness to her beautiful passage and to how the energy medicine that was part of our family held us while we tended the spirit door for her.

Her heavy eyes met mine. It was a struggle for her to lift her head, but I could see that she was still guarding the perimeter of our home and family field. *It's time to rest, girl.* I placed my head against hers. *We'll be okay. You have done such a good job watching over us. Thank you for all that you have done. I love you, Kiva.*

I prepared a spiritual bath and then clarified and blessed the yard. I blessed Kiva's tired body. Once again, I was tending the spirit door by making a sacred space and inviting the presence of spirit to be with us. A gentle breeze ruffled her fur and stirred the branches overhead. Spirit would be here today.

Kiva began the day in the east of the yard, near the front gate and her watchful place. My husband and I spent the hours following her migration through the yard and sitting with her quiet company as the sun moved across the sky. We talked and laughed about our many adventures with her, both before and then with children. In the late afternoon, I watched my children say good-bye to her. Tears washed down my face as they stepped forward one by one, dipping their hands into the spiritual bath and sprinkling Kiva with a final blessing.

My husband drove our children to their aunt and uncle's house. When I was alone with Kiva, I asked how I might find her in the spirit form. Closing my eyes, I let her essence sink deeply into mine. She took her final resting place in the yard. I sensed an energy opening just to the west of her and began to bless this energetic spirit door with blessing water. Soon my husband returned, along with the end-of-life veterinarian we had called to our home.

As an energy reader, I know how to sense the deeper layers of connection between us and the ancestors or spirits of the land. It is something I think we all could do when we were living in the wild, on the earth, bare feet treading on soil. When our breath was shared daily with the cedars and we birthed babies on beds of moss, we certainly knew, even though we likely never pondered, that we were part of a wholeness, a whole continuum of breath and being, vibrating with this life essence, and then the quiet repose of death, an exhale that was meant to occur while lying on the soft earth. And as mothers, we come to know this spirit door in our own body.

And this is why, as I found myself in the August sun near the lavender filled with bees and the grapevines heavy with leaves, I recognized a familiar place. I had come to this spirit door in birthing my three sons and a spirit daughter. The air was expanding and shifting as a soul prepared to make this crossing.

Though the grief lifted me away, I remembered my duty to Kiva; it was our turn to guard the way. I placed both hands around the thick red fur of her neck. My husband sat at her head. She leaned heavily onto my lap. Kiva's last breath came and went. There was a pause, an exhale. And then the energy moved like water, from her body beneath my hands and into the air around us. Her spirit moved across the quiet grass, brushing over my skin, heading west, shining on in the gold light.

A few weeks later, I met Jean Houston, a prominent intuitive. In our brief exchange, she said, "My gift is that I was raised by a dog. I can talk to any dog."

Not expecting this, I reached for her, saying, "I just lost my German shepherd, Kiva. She was the co-mother to my children."

Jean took hold of my hand and asked, "Will you be receiving another German shepherd puppy soon?"

I nodded. *How did she know?*

"Kiva is sending her spirit daughter to you."

Tears filled my eyes.

We found our way to a litter of puppies, born on a small farm south of Portland, in the foothills of the Cascade Range. They were born in August, the day after Kiva's passage. When I came to visit our new puppy, I walked the perimeter of the land with the farm's owner. We passed a mated pair of red Macaws she had kept for forty years. A sense of remembering flooded my being. Just days after Kiva had died, I dreamt of two red Macaws outside my bedroom window.

And so, just as Kiva had come to us many years before, we welcomed her spirit daughter, Moka, to our home. I watched my children respond joyfully to Moka's playful puppy energy. They met her with tenderness and love, and my husband and I witnessed our parenting efforts take hold in their gentle responses. Kiva had cared for these children, and now they were taking care of this pup.

With time and training, Moka would take her full place in the energy of our family. Yet even on the eve of her arrival, I noted that our family energy field once again felt complete. I closed my eyes; everyone gathered in the family bed or in sleeping bags around the soft breath of our new pup. *Thank you, girl*, I whispered to Kiva's spirit.

Tending the spirit door with presence invites us to live fully in our precious lives. Tending the spirit door as a family, we witness the sacredness of life. Following the deeper currents together, we may discover where to reconnect with our own centers and once again remember the way our energy moves like shared breath, along rivers, over fields, like spirits touching down to earth.

A Sacred Life

B efore considering my lineage or even my own path from child-hood, I would first give birth to my sons. Each child called me back to my own center, to the place where the ancient resides. As my days filled with the dreamy play of my children, I searched for the box where I kept my most treasured childhood playthings. It contained three native dolls—all gifts from my maternal grand-mother: one with the fur-lined parka of an Alaskan native; another like a native Hawaiian, with a grass skirt that rustled when you held her; and my favorite—the one with a fringed buckskin dress and thick black hair held by a beaded headband.

Holding the dolls in my hands again, I recalled an event long buried by time. My mother was making costumes for her three daughters to dress as pilgrims in a local parade. To her surprise, I insisted on being a Native American. In an old photo album,

I found the picture of me at six years old, standing with an expression of pure pride in the potato-sack dress and headband that my mom made to satisfy me, her native daughter. In the faded photo, I am there with my sisters in their matching dresses and aprons.

Only now, with the perspective of a mother and a healer, can I appreciate how my play as a child reflected who I was and what I carried. In the rural eastern Washington home of my childhood, I had no reference for native healing ways, but my child essence reached naturally for the dolls that represented this energy current. My life now reflects these dolls. The work I do as a healer, sitting at the spirit door with woman upon woman, is similar to the native medicine used by Maya, Native American, Eskimoan, and other traditional healers—but I could easily have lost my way in the years of schooling that pulled me away from my center.

In mothering and healing, I have found that it is my own center that brings the most potent energy for my life. As my energy skills developed, I felt a strong thread of energy behind me, along the line of my maternal grandfather. We have talked very little, he and I, in the brokenness that family can become, but he eagerly brought photos of his family line when I asked him about his people.

I had a sense of profound recognition when, in one of the photos, I set eyes on the face of my great-great-grandmother, Matilda. She was brown-skinned and bright-eyed, but she also looked somehow displaced, dressed as she was in a stiff dress and corset. Except for the clothes she was wearing, she resembled my dolls. Perhaps she was taken from her people or her traditions but still the energy thread remained—waiting for her great-great-granddaughter to remember her. In another photo, Matilda sits with her husband and five children. The youngest child, my great-grandmother Cora, is on her lap. Matilda would die less than a year later, before Cora turned two.

All that remains of Matilda's story is this: She was born in rural Sweden, married a Norwegian, sailed on a ship to the United States, traveled to Utah, had five children, and died a little more than a year after her last one was born. My great-grandmother Cora had not a single memory of her mother. Yet over the course of her life, she would move in a northern migration pattern, from Utah to Seattle and then to Anchorage, Alaska. She would find her true home, and later die, at the same latitude on the globe as the one where her mother was born.

And her great-great-granddaughter would reawaken to the spirit energy within her hands. She would mother from this place and carry the ancient lineage thread for her sons and grandchildren and great-great-grandchildren to weave into their own sacred lives some day.

You are a blessing, connected to the energy of everything—
may you know this beauty that flows from your own center
as you birth, mother, and live from this place.

Acknowledgments

A book is a baby in that you must set aside your agenda as a writer (or a mother) and receive the unique essence of the creation coming in. My first note of gratitude goes to Beyond Words president and editor in chief, Cynthia Black; Beyond Words publisher, Richard Cohn; and Atria Books publisher, Judith Curr, for their collective ability to hold this work with both precision and the presence of spirit. Heartfelt thanks to their exceptional staff, who midwifed *Mothering from Your Center* with tremendous skill and care: Jenefer Angell, Emily Han, Lindsay S. Brown, Devon Smith, Sheila Ashdown, Jennifer Weaver-Neist, Emmalisa Sparrow, Georgie Lewis, Jessica Sturges, and Whitney Quon.

Profound gratitude to the amazing women who have come to my women's health practice and shared with me the wisdom of the creative center as a resource for mothering, creativity, and life. May you honor your beauty and place in the center so the world can honor you. Thanks to your babies, baby spirits, and other creative inspirations that are bringing in the new potential.

Thanks to my midwife Karen Parker Linn, who sees "the pelvis of a goddess" in every woman and reflects that love in all of her women's care and midwifery practice.

Special thanks to my book club/tribe: Jen, Michelle, Tali, Brooke, Neha, Holly, Mary, and Sara. Together we celebrated our pregnancies and loved the new babies. Our shared laughter at the craziness of this mothering journey keeps me grounded and savoring the blessings.

I give thanks every year for the talented teachers who expand the worlds of our children. This writing year gave our family a gift in that each of our sons had a masterful teacher: Mia Yang, Sarah Rosman, and Michael Jansa. Thank you also to our very special care provider, Sofia Urrutia-Lopez, who is highly creative and spent many hours in imaginary landscapes with our youngest son while I typed away. Gratitude for the musical guidance of Allen Mathews too.

I am thankful to our many family members, who cherish and also nurture our children. Special thanks to my mothering inspirations. My mother, Melodie Petry, gave me the energetic download for cherishing children and recognizing their blessings in our lives. Thanks to my mother-in-law, Janice Kent, for her uncanny ability to see the light in young people and for showing me what I could be by her belief in my potential. To my grandmother Ruth Love. To Julie, for many heart talks. To my father, Glenn Petry, who invited my connection with the land.

Thank you to the gifted healers who helped restore my mothering body and continue to align the energetic field. May every mother have such a team: Joseph Soprani, Sohi McCaw, Liliana Barzola, Marissa Mayer, and Judith Boothby. Special thanks to

Dr. Sheila Murphy for her healing skills, her mothering presence in my life, and for teaching me how to work with babies.

Deep thanks to Amanda Weber-Welch for her beautiful, intuitive presence, time and again. And to her family—Madi, Maya, Bill, and Andrea—for holding our family and youngest son in their warm embrace while we navigated our most serious family health crisis. Special thanks to Mary Frazel and Ron Mariotti for the holistic medicine that brought true healing for our son.

To Nancy Cook and Miss Izi, for the light of the fire that brought in our two babes and for bringing this mothering magic with our solstice children.

To Sara DeLuca, sister of the heart: from late-night excursions to foreign travel, I count this time of mothering as yet another adventure we are so blessed to share together.

Sweet Kiva—my German shepherd co-mother. Thank you for tending this family. Long may your spirit run. Thank you for sending Moka, your spirit daughter. For Blue Magoo and Kona too.

To my eco-hero husband, Dan Kent: What words can I write to the other half of my days? Lover, editor, chef, gardener, best friend, co-parent—your skills in home and life are a perfect balance for us in tending this family and making all things better and brighter. Every day I am glad for you.

And to my beautiful sons—Nick, Gabe, and Japhy. You are the inspiration for all that I am. May you know how to tend the fire that each one of you came in with and discover the purpose of your creative flame. Thank you for inviting me on this mothering path and allowing me space to write. I love you!

To the spirits of the land, my spirit daughter, and the ancestors, I give thanks. Again, deep gratitude to the wild feminine for keeping me company through the dark nights and inspired days, winter and summer, nursing babies and tending children, building a creative motherhood, and whispering words by the fire. You are loved.

Appendix

Women's Stories: In Their Own Words

In working with the healing potential of the female body in thousands of women, there have been so many inspirational stories. The stories are what have moved me to write books and share the extraordinary medicine we carry in our bodies as women. I wish that all the stories could be told, but here are a few that crossed my path in the last few months of writing *Mothering from Your Center*. These narratives detail some difficult times. Though we often prefer ease, every mother will encounter places of challenge on her journey, if not through conception or birth then with lineage issues, partner conflicts, illnesses, or even the routine stresses of mothering. These stories reveal that in meeting the hardships with presence, we may also find our greatest potential. I invited the women to tell their stories in their own words.

I am a small-business owner, married with two children. There is a constant dance of time—enough time to put into my paid work and unpaid work, enough time to enjoy my kids and husband and express my love for all of them, and enough time for myself. In my mother's generation, it was a battle. A fight for women's rights and equality. A struggle to make it in a man's world. That corporate climb no longer exists. The energy of struggle creates stagnation and conflict.

After working with Tami as a healer and then studying with her as a practitioner, I began to approach my life from a feminine perspective—that is, from a place of nurturing and circular thinking. Now I use the energy of my pelvic bowl to move forward and make clear boundaries. The flow of money, the safety of our home, the mothering and marriage— it all comes from my center. The pelvic bowl brings a softer, deeper, and stronger energy to the balance of my life.

My bowl is a precious gift, a private pearl that I cherish and protect. I am blessed to be able to work with women as a practitioner, too, helping them access the energy of their own bowl. In doing such work, it is a constant reinforcement of the role that it plays in every woman's life. I see the power of release—emotionally, physically, and energetically—and the impact of such movement from the center. It translates to decision making about marriage and divorce, shifting careers, conceiving a child, or healing from a loss. Once the bowl is cleared, the clarity and relief on the woman's face is so apparent. She is lighter, clearer in her choices, and able to manifest something far beyond her reach.

—*Beth, acupuncturist, owner of Mississippi Health Center,*
and mother of two

Prior to my second cesarean for placenta previa, I discovered *Wild Feminine*. With no option for a natural birth, I was feeling disheartened. Tami's words brought me back into my body and connected me with my baby. I corresponded with Tami. She encouraged me to tell my baby and my body what was about to happen prior to the cesarean. I went in feeling calm. During the cesarean, I focused on moving birth energy out of my vagina as they were pushing my daughter into the world. It was a lovely experience. It was not my ideal, but it was lovely.

Six weeks later, I met Tami, and she introduced me to the power of my birth energy. We had a lovely session, where I was able to rebirth both of my children. I energetically delivered them in a space where I wanted to be and with the people I wanted around me. Amazingly, this space never would have been a reality under any circumstance, so the birth experience was more beautiful than I could have imagined. I went home feeling lighter and freer than I had in two years. And I released tissue and fluid, emotion and disappointment.

I rebirthed my children several times over the next several days. And after a few weeks, I was at peace. I don't think about my births with sadness anymore. I celebrate my scars. I'm no longer ashamed and no longer hide them from my husband and bodyworkers. They are a part of me. I show them to my children and tell them how they came into this world. I tap into this powerful energy to carry myself and my children through our days. I've noticed that when I focus on my birth energy for myself or my children, we are all able to go with the flow more easily.

—Kate, mother and horse lover

My birth was not the romantic, sacred event that my partner and I had hoped for. The transport from home and unexpected cesarean felt traumatic, frightening, and immense. Internally, I felt great amounts of pain and postpartum anxiety. My body's recovery was very slow. The cesarean surgery disconnected the top of my body from my bottom, and I felt my pelvis haunted by the ghosts of my birth. The labor I experienced was left without finish, a child pulled from my womb mid-transition. This feeling became locked inside my pelvic bowl. I had a difficult time connecting with myself or accepting or exploring my interior along with my exterior.

Eleven months after my birth, I went to see Tami. The first appointment I had was the most opening and connecting experience I have had with my body since before the pregnancy. I literally watched the anxiety float out of my life. The birthing energy felt warm and healing, repairing and attentive. While smoothing out muscle knots, thinning scar tissue, restructuring bones, and balancing my pelvic bowl, the three sessions with Tami called in the birthing energy I did not have, offering me the support one year postpartum to truly heal from my birth.

—Alissa, artist, landscape contractor, and mama

I planned a home birth. I prepared with herbs, candles, soft music, chiropractic adjustments, acupuncture treatments, rituals, and a circle of support. My labor stalled, or my cervix failed to progress, or my baby was stuck, or I wasn't as ready as I thought I was. I did not plan a seventy-two-hour labor, transfer to the hospital, cascading medical interventions, and eventual C-section birth—but that's what I got. I fought my way out of the hospital with a profound sense of failure and distrust in my body. I was a failure. I was given the gift, the responsibility of mothering this tiny, perfect creature, and I failed. On my first day! I felt profoundly alone. I was utterly in love with my daughter and yet full of fear that something terrible was going to happen to her, that I wouldn't be able to stop her suffering. I normalized all these terrible feelings and battled the new moments and months of parenthood from that place.

I came to see Tami eighteen months after my daughter was born, and I said, "I'm still pregnant. I didn't get to give birth!" Tami released grief and fear from me physically without retraumatizing me. But the most profound thing was the sense of connecting my energetic womb-love to my child. I felt an eternity of sparkly light—brighter than sunshine—pour out of me, out of my incision site (!), to my darling daughter. The sense of this connection as real was more profound than my previous sense of failure. Almost instantly, I felt more myself and confident in my mothering. I confronted, with Tami's help, my fear that the world wasn't a safe place. And I sank into the newly discovered knowledge that my womb is not just safe but profoundly nurturing, and that energetically this safety is accessible to my daughter and me at all times.

Within days, I noticed myself occupying my body and the world more comfortably. The story of my daughter's birth began to lose its control over me and blend into the landscape, rich in stories of motherhood. I slowly began to feel not like a failure but triumphant and brave for having worked so hard and surviving surgery with some resilience. And for the first time, I allowed my mothering love in fully. I understood, in my body, what it is to love like a mother, with generations of mothers beside me. My daughter responded in kind. We walk the path solidly together now.

—*Sue, mother, feminist, swimmer,*
and herbalist

Post-birth, I never experienced the rush of "happy" hormones I'd heard about. I worried incessantly about the health of my son and was sure that the birth itself—an unexpected breech home birth with an initially unconscious baby—was the cause of his allergies and inability to sleep longer than forty-five minutes. It took two and half years for my son to finally start sleeping for longer periods. That's when the dark cloud began to lift, but the guilt and regret about his birth still hung on tightly.

This year (my son is now ten), two people suggested that I try internal massage with Tami. I read her book *Wild Feminine* prior to the session. During the massage, she had me envision going back to before labor started. I imagined sitting in my peaceful living room with the light streaming in the beautiful old windows. I put my hands on my belly and talked to and loved that little baby inside me. She then had me imagine holding my son after he was out, safe and healthy. I pictured nursing him and seeing his precious little body nestled against mine.

Both Tami and I could feel a shift happen. She said it was the birth energy opening up. As I cried, I felt a peace settle over the memories that had previously caused pain. When I left her office, I could feel that open energy. I remembered it post-birth, a very open sensitivity. It was like there were no barriers between me and everything in the world. I felt like I needed to be careful about what stimuli I allowed around me. There was joy but also vulnerability. I noticed something had lifted, perhaps the disappointment or regret around my birth experience. I felt like it was all okay. I was okay. My son was okay. There was a calmness there that I hadn't realized had been missing. Even the love I felt for my son felt easier and lighter.

When I picked him up from school later that day, something between he and I had shifted. I could see him separately from myself. I could see his humor and gentle disposition from another perspective. I could see that he was okay and that I didn't need to worry about him anymore. And even though I thought we already had a close relationship, I felt a new intimacy, a clearer connection between us. Since then, I often go back to those images, holding my belly before his birth and holding him afterward when he was safe. It brings much peace, and I can feel that birth energy open again. I often take that energy to the present day when I'm holding my healthy, happy ten-year-old in my arms. It is a blessing to have access to that.

—*Annalee, mother, accountant, yogi,*
and trapeze enthusiast

My belief was certain: I did not want to be a mother. All the women in my family—my mother, aunts, grandmother, great-grandmothers (on both sides)—struggled as mothers.

Motherhood was unsafe terrain. It meant a life of unfulfilled dreams. I was more than willing to give away my feminine center and fill it with all the masculinity (i.e., power and control) I could muster. I was determined to be different, to be better.

When I arrived in Portland for a Holistic Pelvic Care (HPC) provider training with Tami, I had spent years working to heal that belief system. My partner, new baby boy, and stepdaughter traveled with me as testament to that healing and my mothering. Yet as I listened to Tami speak about the power of the mother, I began to understand the deeper healing work that remained. Instead of carrying wounds, I wanted to reconnect to the medicine of my body.

When I started the HPC training, the first realization in my bowl was an awareness of the only power I had ever connected to my feminine center: giving birth. The mothering gene may have skipped our family, but the birthing gene had not. Never for one second had I doubted my ability to give birth. This was a connection to my mother. She had also had good births. Thinking about it now, birthing was the most comfortable space we have shared as mother and daughter.

Receiving pelvic work called upon these simple truths. It also called to mind my son's birth. By all standards his birth had been perfect. However, there was a moment of knowing in my body and spirit that something wasn't working. Touching the physical place now brought it to clarity: I was still afraid of mothering. After three days of intensive work in the class, my pelvic bowl was feeling strong and grounded. There was a resonance in my center—perhaps more resonance than there had ever been. Still, I had unequal body and pelvic sensations. I was easily fatigued on the right side and had a difficult time sensing through the left side. Tami invited me to explore this imbalance with an energy session.

Before we began the session, I shared with Tami something I had held back: When I was eighteen I had a daughter. From the moment her spirit entered my body, I was sure that she belonged to someone else. Releasing her in an open adoption felt like the only way to honor that truth. It was also the way I believed I could save her from the patterns of our history. Her thirteenth birthday was on that very day I met with Tami.

Receiving this information as sacred and beautiful, Tami placed her hand over my womb space. I felt a swell of warmth from the inside. Though I was sure I would find laughter and joy in the treatment, the bowl always tells the truth, so with the swell came tears and sadness. The tears weren't fresh; they were old. Tami asked if I could identify what was happening. Yes; I had denied my daughter. I had hoped to prevent giving her the scars I carried, but instead I had given her different ones. I felt regret and guilt and sadness for the wound I had given her.

Tami spoke a truth about mothering: "We do the best we can, but sometimes we scar them." She continued as a palpable energy pulsed and bounded out of my body, "We do our healing work so that they can do theirs. We can mother and give love to our children even when they are not present with us. We can connect to them through the root and give blessings."

She encouraged me to visualize this experience. I felt warmth flow from my root into somewhere in the distance and back through the top of my womb space. I felt connection and love.

Tami brought my focus to my left ovary. It was empty. This feminine space had no definition, but how could she when I had never given her any? Frustration and anger washed over me. Tami helped me guide my breath to the area and define the frustration. I was shocked to find flashes of my stepdaughter and the too-frequent moments I disconnected from her, quieted her voice, or controlled her expression. A flood of words and emotions came through. Caring for this child as if she were my own, yet not feeling like that is allowed. A dynamic child with a creative, bold voice, her curiosity matches my own and triggers me. She wants to connect; she is everywhere I am, like a shadow. (My mom used to call me her shadow.) I am afraid to connect. I am afraid to hurt her. I am afraid to connect to her and to lose her.

Tami lowered her voice and spoke to me softly with instructive intention. I don't recall her exact words, but I know they gave me permission to mother all my children.

By the end of the session I had experienced mother healing on every level: healing the mother line and the inner child, healing birth events, giving energy blessings to children even when they are not directly with us, and balancing birth and stepchildren. I felt peace for the first time in far too long. I came to understand that mothering is holding and releasing; it is fluid and formless. Tami encouraged me to release my historical experience of mothering and to reclaim my territory. She showed me that this is the path of mothering from the center.

—*Kristin, women's health practitioner*
and mother

On a quiet morning in early April 2006, I held my five-year-old son, Cameron, in my arms as he took his final breath. After a four-year battle with cancer, his body could take no more. In his final weeks on this earth, his little body was wracked with so much pain that he was unable to walk, let alone even sit on the floor to play. My vibrant little boy deteriorated before my eyes, and I felt utterly and completely helpless.

My instinct and desire to mother was still there, yet my child was gone. There were no more little clothes to launder, precious hands to hold, silly songs to sing, or adventures to take together. I felt like a part of me had been torn away. With Cameron gone, I could no longer identify with myself as a mother, and this was yet another deep loss that began to engrain in my spirit.

This past year, as a third-year naturopathic medical student, I took a four-day intensive seminar, taught by Tami, to be trained in Holistic Pelvic Care. I arrived at the seminar anxious to learn this therapy as a modality for my future medical practice. During the second day of training, I realized this therapy would be crucial to any woman like me, who had suffered through the loss of a child. As we talked about energetic holding patterns in the pelvic bowl and the physical changes that could occur to the pelvic organs, musculature, and fascia as a result of grief, loss, or unresolved emotions, I wondered how much my own connection to my feminine might have been affected by the loss of my son.

That evening, Tami offered to do a session with me, and I agreed. As the session began, I could feel the years of sorrow, suppression, and loss building like a giant wave. I had a clear vision of a stressful day in the hospital; my son was only three at the time. I recalled the oncologist giving me terrible news that the cancer had spread, this time to Cameron's brain. I remember struggling not to cry and holding it together as I always did, so as not to scare or trouble my son.

I began to sob, releasing the many years of pain and struggle that I had not allowed myself to feel. Deep in my pelvic bowl, I felt a hot, burning tightness that slowly dispelled and melted away under Tami's touch. With this, I found a relief and lightness in my body I had not felt in years.

I was deeply exhausted for two days following my session with Tami, yet I felt a connection with myself that I had never really recognized. As I reflected on both the training and personal session, I realized something quite beautiful and profound. The simplicity in reconnecting with my feminine reminded me that I am still a mother—that I will always be a mother. That role is a part of me, inherent in my feminine lineage and accessible to all women regardless of whether they have children or not. While I may no longer have my son to physically nurture, my connection to him is not lost. By connecting to my feminine energy and grounding myself to the earth, I am able to connect to the very first place that ever nurtured my son—my feminine, my womb.

—*Michelle, naturopathic medical student and spirit mother*

An Unexpected Hospital Stay

When this book was moving into the final editing stages, my youngest son, four-year-old Japhy, had a sudden belly pain that necessitated emergency surgery for a ruptured appendix. We spent two very intense weeks in the hospital, corresponding with his fifth birthday. As I watched my home-birthed child go into surgery and endure many medical processes, I called on spirit to hold us both. I stayed by Japhy's side through days and nights of seemingly endless pain that were the path to his recovery. It was surreal to be lying with him wrapped in my arms, in the hospital bed on his birthday—as if it were a hospital birth five years after being born. I slept in his bed, massaged his legs, and literally wrapped my body around his to let our energy connection bring healing. I also entered his world of play to help him navigate the pain and medical procedures—dragons, unicorns, and superheroes surrounded us at all times. And though my husband was there each day to help and hold us both, like birth, it felt that there was a point where my son and I traveled this path, just he and I.

As I faced my own fears in holding a gravely ill child, Michelle's words from the previous story came to mind; I remembered her courage. If you are in a difficult place as a mother, chances are there is another mother who has traveled there as well. We are stronger when we place our mothering hearts together.

I also called upon holistic medicine to support the healing that would continue for many months—homeopathics from our naturopath in the hospital and then twice daily vitamin-filled smoothies (see page 282 for the recipe) after returning home; energy work to restore energy balance and clear the trauma of the procedures that, while life-saving, were only perceived as hurtful by our young son; bodywork and acupressure to restore whole body flow and recover from the surgery; summer days of raspberry picking and walking barefoot for renewed energy from the land; space for the entire family's pent-up emotional expression and recalibration, and extra doses of sleep with a solid stream of laughter, hugs, and love.

In a hospital stay or with any prolonged illness or injury, use your wild mothering resources: make a spiritual bath (or have one made for you) and bless the hospital room—and your child—morning and night; call upon the Great Mother to hold you; drop into pure presence and play with your child; send your child energy with the birth energy meditation whenever you are apart, or for any medical procedures. I felt my son's energy come to me while he was in surgery and had an image of him climbing into my lap to nurse—the connection between mother and child is profound and powerful. This connection can be called upon to assist these most difficult situations by meditating on the vibrant birth flow between you and your child.

Take care of yourself as well. Balance your energy with the Pelvic Bowl Sings exercise (page 248); ask for and receive the support you need; and remember the healing potential contained simply within your touch and presence. Listen to the intuitive response from your center, even in the midst of the medical process and the authority of medical providers. Your intuition has essential guidance and medicine because you are a mother. Rest into your bond with your child and the life-giving river of birth energy. Let this flow energize the beauty of such pure time spent together.

Japhy's Power Berry Smoothie

- ½ to ¾ cup fresh or frozen raspberries or blueberries (If frozen, warm some of the berries so the smoothie is not ice cold, this aids digestion.)
- ¼ cup yogurt
- ⅓ cup coconut milk or almond milk
- 1 heaping Tbsp ground flax seeds
- 1 packet (1000 mg) raspberry Emergen-C
- 1 tsp (300–500 mg) buffered vitamin C
- ½ tsp probiotic powder
- 5 drops ChlorOxygen (concentrated chlorophyll from nettles)
- optional: 1 Tbsp whey powder (omit for dairy sensitivity) and/or a dash of cinnamon

Blend ingredients and enjoy!

Affirmations for Inspired Mothering

One of the most common challenges I hear from the mothers in my women's health practice is that they are lonely. Mothering can feel like so much giving with too little received in return. The antidote to this is gathering with other women and mothers. Though difficult to navigate with busy lives and hectic schedules, a routine commitment to gather with women friends is essential.

My longtime book club—my tribe of mothers—has been gold for me and my mothering. I asked them to come up with a sentence or two that distilled what they had learned so far in mothering. These nine women became mothers together and now have twenty-five children among them. This is what they shared:

> Though the world offers many opinions, your mother's intuition is golden. Also, don't be afraid to learn from your children.

> You are your child's best advocate. You are also your own best advocate.

> It is okay to ask for help—from your children, partner, family and friends, the universe. Then when our children need support, they will know it is okay for them to ask for it.

> Let go when you need to or are able to, as this shall pass. Each day savor the blessings, because this, too, will pass.

> Mothering has its own seasonal rhythm. Embrace the wonderful and the challenge, since all of it will shift and bring a whole new landscape in the mothering journey.

Try not to compare yourself to your mothering friends. The choices you make for your child will be the right ones for you.

Experience helps you find your own parenting style; being true to that is essential.

Breathe. Breathe. Breathe. Did I mention breathe?

Take the time to be childish with your kids. Skip, jump, be silly, have cake for breakfast . . . it is much easier than being a grown-up.

When your kids are grumpy or at their most challenging, don't take it personally, because it isn't personal.

Focus your attention on the connection between you and your child. Let go of the details and move toward whatever strengthens this connection.

Love yourself as much as you love your children.

Find your mothering tribe.

May you and your mothering be blessed.

List of Exercises

Resources for Finding a Pelvic Care Practitioner

Women's pelvic care can assist postpartum healing, promote general global wellness, and help prevent long-term pelvic problems. To find a pelvic care practitioner:

- Visit www.wildfeminine.com to find more information about my own Holistic Pelvic Care practice as well as a growing list of Holistic Pelvic Care providers.
- Call your local physical therapy clinic to inquire about a women's health physical therapist on staff. Interview any potential providers. Ask if they use vaginal massage in their treatment practice (because not all women's health physical therapists are trained in internal techniques). Ask about the types of pelvic conditions they treat. Practitioners who treat pelvic pain (as opposed to just incontinence) often have the most advanced manual (hands-on) skills.
- Find a local practitioner of the Arvigo Techniques of Maya Abdominal Therapy. This technique, developed by naprapathic physician and herbalist Dr. Rosita Arvigo and based on traditional healing methods of Maya medicine, addresses pelvic flow and organ alignment through abdominal and sacral massage, for both women and men.
- Through the Barral Institute, find a local practitioner trained in abdominal or pelvic visceral massage (massage of the abdominal or pelvic organs). These techniques, developed by French osteopath Dr. Jean-Pierre Barral, also address core alignment and flow for both women and men.

Take good care of your sacred center.
May the beauty shine. May the bowl sing.